Successful Case Management in Long-Term Care

Joan Quinn, RN, MSN, FAAN, is president of Connecticut Community Care, Inc., and Community Care Network of Connecticut, Inc. She is the past Executive Director of Triage, Inc., a nationally recognized community-based health research and demonstration program. She is a committee member for the Public/Private Partnership for Financing Long-Term Care for the Elderly. She is a consultant to the Governor's Commission on Long-Term Care for the Elderly in Connecticut, as well as to The Travelers Insurance Companies, Aetna, and Blue Cross/ Blue Shield of Connecticut and New Jersey regarding long-term care insurance product development and case management in long-term care. She has received the American Nurses' Association Gerontological Nurse of the Year Award and is a Fellow of the American Academy of Nursing. She is the author of numerous publications and serves as editorial advisor for several professional journals. She has lectured and consulted nationally on long-term care issues and the role of care management, and has testified before Congress on topics such as financing of long-term care, home and community-based services for the elderly, and case management.

Successful Case Management in Long-Term Care

Joan Quinn, RN, MSN, FAAN

Springer Publishing Company • New York

Springer Publishing Company, Inc.
536 Broadway
New York, NY 10012-3955

93 94 95 96 97 / 5 4 3 2 1

Library of Congress Cataloging-in-Publication Data

Quinn, Joan.
Successful case management in long-term care / Joan Quinn.
p. cm.
Includes bibliographical references and index.
ISBN 0-8261-7750-6
1. Aged—Long-term care. 2. Long-term care of the sick.
3. Handicapped—Long-term care. 4. Continuum of care.
5. Medical social work. I. Title.
[DNLM: 1. Delivery of Health Care—United States. 2. Long-Term Care—methods. 3. Long-Term Care—organization & administration. 4. Patient Care Planning—methods. 5. Patient Care Planning—organization & administration. W 84.7 Q7s]
RA564.8.Q56 1993
362.1'6—dc20
DNLM/DLC
for Library of Congress 92-49033
CIP

Printed in the United States of America

Contents

Foreword

Many people can and, fortunately, do live into their later years in reasonably good health and independence. Nevertheless, it is clear that more and more families will face situations in which an older member has developed complex medical problems, with variable degrees of loss of independence and need for assistance. For these people, working out a sound, comprehensive, supportive approach to meeting the care needs may seem almost impossible. Furthermore, the types of services needed will very likely change over time and adjustments will need to be made, calling upon a variety of resources related to health care, including both social and financial. Very few persons have the knowledge and experience to manage such complexities on their own.

It is to meet such challenges that the growing field of case management services has been rapidly developing. Starting with such pioneering efforts as those of the author of this book and her imaginative program of community care, Ms. Quinn and others in this country and elsewhere have developed and demonstrated the great value of trained and experienced professionals in the fields of health and social services. One of the most promising developments from these efforts is the very individualized approach to meeting the care needs of persons with complex, difficult problems.

Successful case management involves, first of all, a thorough, comprehensive evaluation of the medical, functional, and social problems present, followed by the development of a plan of care. The next step is to identify and help make arrangements for the various resources required to meet the needs of the affected person and her or his family. The value of this approach has now been amply demonstrated in many settings.

It is indeed timely that this guide to case management has been prepared as a further step in extending the use of sound principles and approaches to the benefit of many more people.

T. Franklin Williams, MD

Acknowledgments

Over the past 15 years, the federal and state governments have grappled with the growing numbers of elderly and disabled persons with long-term care needs. The health care system has not been well developed to target this group of people, as its primary focus has been on acute, short-term services. In the 1970s, the federal government, concerned both with these growing population groups and the escalating costs of care, funded waiver programs across the country. These programs had a key service component, case management.

As time passed after the start of the early demonstrations, case management became the "hot topic" and "buzz word" of the late 1980s and continues to be to the present time. However, if you have seen "one case management agency," you have seen "one case management agency." The definition of the service and the qualifications of the staff often differ dramatically across sites.

Concern about the uneven quality of agencies and their case management functions motivated the publishing of this book. It is designed to assist new and existing case managers and case management organizations with their important work. The case manager's professionalism, advocacy, and sensitivity to clients, families, and the formal providers of care is essential to successful interventions and outcomes for the clients and families.

Chapters of this book were written using the expertise of professionals with many years of case management and organizational experience. A number of colleagues have assisted with content, gathering literature, reviewing assessment materials, and by speaking with other peers.

Special acknowledgment is given to Jean Burton, MSW, who worked diligently in the development of this manuscript over the past nine months.

Special gratitude is expressed to Myra Kerr, RN, MS, director of quality assurance at Connecticut Community Care, Inc. for her review and rewrites.

Appreciation is given also to Cheryl Whitman, RN, MS, director of educational services at Connecticut Community Care, Inc.; Diane Bock, RN, BS, case manager and case manager supervisor at Connecticut Community Care, Inc.; and, Jane Birk, RN, BSN, an employee for many years at Triage, Inc. and of Connecticut Community Care, Inc.

Finally, thanks to Ferne Waskowicz, my executive assistant, who provided her expert skill in the editing and typing of this book.

NOTE: Although this publication uses "she" to describe the client and/or case manager, "he" is also intended.

1 What Is Case Management Anyway?

Dora and Sam live in their own home. Dora helps Sam with dressing and bathing, because Sam has emphysema and severe arthritis. One day, while assisting Sam, Dora slips, falls, and breaks her hip. Sam calls his daughter who lives nearby for help. She tells him to call 911 immediately. After emergency and corrective treatment in the hospital, Dora returns home with instructions that she will be called by a Case Management Agency to continue her rehabilitation (Connecticut Community Care, Inc., 1991).

Dora and Sam are about to enter the formal world of long-term care. They could be facing one of the most confusing and exhausting experiences of *their* lives. Or, they might have a relatively easy journey negotiating this new territory, because they will hire a seasoned guide. Whatever the outcome, Dora and Sam will be joining a growing number of people with problems and needs similar to their own.

Long-term care case management is designed for people like Dora and Sam who will require different types of care over an extended period of time. As their care needs change, these individuals will move further into the long-term care system, a combination of health and social services offered in institutional, community, or in-home settings, to find suitable services. Public policy planners and health planners alike envision this system as a continuum of care, a range of services ranging from the acute care hospital to the nursing home with 24-hour skilled nursing services, and on into the community and in-home services for supportive or maintenance care. Provision of all of these types of services is influenced by who pays for the service, where it is delivered, and what is available to assist fragile, disabled persons. Case management services are focused toward helping dependent individuals through the care system. If the system indeed works as planned, Dora and Sam will maintain their independence in their own home by securing assistance from many care providers with the guidance of a knowledgeable case manager.

The majority of persons requiring some type of long-term care are old-old, those 75 years of age and older. However, there is a growing number of younger individuals who also need health or social services to help manage their lives. Persons of any age can suffer functional impairments or mental and physical disabilities; they can contract acquired immunodeficiency syndrome (AIDS) with its debilitating effects; they can experience a traumatic injury that leads to a long-term disability; or, they can have a congenital defect that results in the need for long-term care services. Part of growing old, however, may be learning how to live with the gradual onset of chronic conditions—not life threatening, but disabling in some way. These limitations are a normal risk of aging, and in this society, where life expectancy reaches into the 75 years plus range, they are to be anticipated and can even be planned for both in the public sector and privately. By incorporating this dual perspective, the long-term care system can become a benefit to those persons in need. The available services can improve the quality of life and the sense of well-being for impaired individuals, including the frail elderly.

THE FUNDAMENTALS OF CASE MANAGEMENT

When the Case Management Agency called Dora, she needed immediate help and also continued services to assist her disabled husband while she was recuperating. Their daughter took care of Sam's needs while Dora was hospitalized, but the daughter could not provide care to both parents. Dora was told she needs a case manager, but she does not know what that is! (Connecticut Community Care, Inc., 1991).

Case management has been called many things and defined in many ways. It is not case management, it is care management, because it is the care, not the case that requires managing. It is not care management, it is care assistance, because the clients need help in managing their own care. It has also been called case coordination, service coordination, service management, service monitoring, and others. This author believes that case management for long-term care is based on three tenets: it is a *holistic approach* to the client; it is a *problem-solving strategy* for the client; and, it is a *dynamic process* involving the interactions among the case manager, the client, and the providers of care (including the family and other informal supporters, formal agencies, and physicians, if necessary). Considering the imperfect state of the long-term care service delivery system, case management can be an invaluable means for disabled persons to gain access to crucial care.

In the holistic approach, the case manager performs a comprehensive assessment of the individual's condition by exploring all aspects of the client's living situation. The case manager gathers information on the client's health, emotional status, cognitive abilities, functional levels, support system, environment, and financial situation. This information is needed for the case manager to gain a holistic understanding of the client and to develop an effective set of goals and objectives for care specifically tailored to each client.

The second fundamental tenet of case management is that it is a problem-solving strategy, developed in collaboration with the client and the family. Once the information gathering process is completed, the case manager and client can discuss the client's strengths and problem areas, and begin to work out appropriate solutions. While the client and/or family may identify several problems, they probably are not aware of possible other problems or solutions. The case manager can help by clearly defining the problem for them, suggesting alternative strategies for coping with each issue, and guiding them toward the decisions that will resolve the problems. Critical to this process, however, is the case manager's "management role." By involving the client and family in the problem discussion and resolution, the case manager maintains the objectivity necessary to help the client make an informed decision about her care needs. For instance, Dora's broken hip made it impossible for her to cook on the days that her daughter did not visit the couple. To the relief of the daughter, who might have lost her job if she had been needed to come every day, the case manager suggested supplementing the daughter's help with meals-on-wheels on alternate days until Dora recovered enough to resume cooking unaided. In the full sense, case management becomes a method both for identifying existing problems and also anticipating future problems and preparing for them.

Finally, case management is by nature a dynamic process. After contacting the client, analyzing the assessment information, and developing problem-solving strategies, the case manager must ensure that client decisions are translated into an effective plan of care. The case manager negotiates with the appropriate service providers in the community and arranges for the services to be delivered as planned. Here, the case manager must both manage the client's services and act as the intermediary between the client and the provider agencies. The client's needs frequently change over time. For example, the client's condition may worsen, providers may discontinue a service, the client may be dissatisfied with a particular provider, or a family member who had been helping out with shopping moves, leaving a gap in the client's care. In most cases, the case manager must find creative ways to finance a client's care plan, through both traditional and nontraditional sources. Perhaps this means accessing a little-known community fund to pay for chore services, or helping the client file for veteran's benefits, or reimbursing a neighbor for gas money to transport the client to the grocery store. To the case manager, these challenges create the dynamism of case management clinical practice. Immersed in the interaction between the client, family, and providers, the case manager must manage the care through the constant integration of informal and formal services. The manager's goals are to be aware of changes as they occur in the client's situation and to maintain an ongoing relationship among the client, the family, and the service provider network.

In the literature, case management has been referred to as a broker of services, similar to an insurance agent or stock broker. The case manager fulfills this function, but only as one part of a greater role. For example, Dora receives a home health aide three times a week to help bathe Sam. After a few weeks, the home health aide arrives very late or even skips a visit. Dora is upset, but she is reluctant to speak out to the aide when she does arrive for fear the aide might be careless with Sam, or even not come to care for Sam any longer. When the case manager calls about something unrelated, Dora mentions this worry. The case manager contacts the provider agency and talks to the aide's supervisor. After speaking with the aide, the supervisor discovers that the aide has a sick son and has been taking him to the clinic lately, but having no vacation time left, she did not mention it to the agency. The supervisor changes her schedule to incorporate the clinic visits and the aide resumes normal hours at Dora's. Thus, the case manager acted on the client's behalf to resolve the service problem and, as a result, became better acquainted with the agency personnel and developed more confidence in the agency's overall services. This dynamic process energizes the long-term care system: the continuous interaction between individuals and the variety of community and institutional services, with the case manager bringing an understanding of how everyone can work together to meet the client's needs.

THE STEPS OF CASE MANAGEMENT

For the case manager and the client receiving the service, the case management process is divided into different steps. Each step is based upon the one before, building a practical and sound approach to the problems at hand. To introduce the elements of case management, a brief description of each component is presented.

Referral and Prescreening

Referral and prescreening are the first steps in the process. At this point, information is obtained about the person to determine whether or not case management is needed. If not, the person should be referred to other resources in the community. If the person's profile appears suitable for case management, then she can be evaluated through the full assessment process.

Assessment

Assessment further confirms the person's appropriateness for case management through a comprehensive collection and analysis of personal information. Because a full evaluation of a person's situation requires the knowledge of health and social professionals, assessment information is usually reviewed by a multidisciplinary team at the outset, or other professionals are consulted before the final evaluation is completed. Professionals involved in this phase can be nurses, social workers, physicians, mental health professionals, nurse practitioners, nutritionists, oral health specialists, pharmacists, or rehabilitative therapists. During the assessment, the following areas are examined.

Health: current and past medical conditions, symptoms,

medications taken, vision and hearing capabilities, and communication ability are evaluated. Also, the client's self-perception of her health is determined.

Emotional status: the client's feelings, social functioning, and behavior are elicited.

Cognitive abilities: these are measured by questioning the client to determine her mental status and ability to reason and make judgements.

Functional abilities: these are measured by determining the client's ability to perform personal care tasks and manage household activities.

Support system: this is evaluated by learning about the client's support or helping network of family and friends by finding out who helps them now and what kinds of assistance she receives. The case manager often corroborates this information with the designated supporters. For example, Sam's daughter came three times each week to do laundry, clean the house, and cook a meal for her parents.

Environment: this is evaluated by examining the home and living situation for hazards and suitability to the client's level of mobility. For instance, are stairs impossible for Dora to climb with her broken hip? Or is the bathroom unsafe for Sam to bathe? Is there any equipment available that would enhance their functioning?

Financial status: this is evaluated by determining the client's income, assets, and expenses and reviewing her eligibility for any entitlement programs. For example, would Dora and Sam qualify for food stamps or are they receiving all Medicare benefits for which they are eligible?

All of this data is then analyzed and problems and resources are identified in preparation for the next step.

Care Planning

Care planning is the next step in the case management process. Having identified the strengths and problems of the client during the assessment process, the case manager works with the client and her caregivers to develop a care plan. This plan outlines all of the details about the services to be provided: the amount, the duration, the times of scheduled services, the providers, which can be either family and friends (informal providers) or community agencies (formal providers), payment sources, and, most important, the responsibilities of all of the persons involved in the caregiving process.

Service Coordination, Delivery, and Reimbursement

Service coordination, service delivery, and service reimbursement are primary responsibilities of the case manager. In this step, the case manager arranges for the actual delivery of services defined in the care plan. For this task, the case manager must have a thorough and current knowledge of community resources in order to select the most appropriate service provider(s) for the client. Appropriateness here denotes quality of service, reasonable cost, and efficient delivery of service. The service reimbursement function varies among care management organizations. For example, a case manager operating out of a Social/Health Maintenance Organization may have greater authority over financial resources than a case manager in an independent case management agency. This degree of authority over service funds can determine the boundaries of a case manager's influence, and affect the design of the care plan and the selection of service providers.

Monitoring

Monitoring is the next component of the case management process. Oncc the care plan is in place, the case manager must maintain a regular schedule of contact with the client and providers of service to ensure the continued appropriateness of the client's care plan. The case manager verifies that services are being delivered as ordered and as needed by the client. In this monitoring phase, case managers must keep informed of the client's situation, adjusting the levels of service as indicated to achieve the most effective use of resources and the highest quality of life for the client. Monitoring challenges the expertise of case managers to maintain a reliable integration of information and services in sometimes very complex circumstances.

Reassessment

Reassessment completes the loop of the case management process. The case manager first reevaluates the initial baseline assessment and subsequent changes. On a regular basis, the case manager conducts a formal, thorough review of the client's status to ascertain whether any changes have occurred in the client's situation or level of functioning. This step includes reevaluating the goals established in the initial care plan. Services are reviewed and revised as necessary. However, at any time, as changes occur in the client's status, the case manager will adjust the care plan accordingly. Regular reassessment ensures that an updated, comprehensive profile of the client is maintained.

Case management service is an important component of the long-term care service system. This service has evolved in response to an imperfect system and is used as a means to integrate and coordinate a variety of existing services. Case management serves the clients by negotiating the system and organizing the jumble of providers, services, and funding sources to meet each client's unique needs.

The remaining chapters of this book provide a guide to the specific components of the case management process.

The next chapter gives an overview of the long-term care delivery system and its continuing evolution, including case management.

A detailed discussion of assessment and care planning is provided in Chapters 3 and 4. Chapter 5 focuses on special care planning issues. Monitoring and evaluation are explored in Chapter 6. Chapter 7 presents a summary of case management models and recommendations concerning staff qualifications and supervision.

2 Overview of the Long-Term Care Delivery System

One of the privileges of living in the 20th century has been to witness the miracles taking place in health care. Medical technologies have developed vaccines to prevent previously devastating diseases such as polio, smallpox, and diphtheria, and medications to greatly reduce deaths from infections such as pneumonia, influenza, meningitis, and others. Modern medicine has an impressive arsenal of high-technology equipment for diagnostic and treatment purposes, and includes new drug treatments to stave off the crippling effects of arthritis, high blood pressure, and heart and other diseases. Scientific research has helped to improve agricultural techniques that increase crop yields, providing food for more people. Better sanitation methods have contributed to a healthier environment. The interest in health promotion and disease prevention have been recognized by many people. As a result, individuals live longer and more healthful lives. Men and women can expect to live well into their 70s and beyond.

Longer life, however, may mean increased vulnerability to and risk of developing chronic, incurable conditions, some associated with aging. These afflictions may include heart disease, osteoporosis, hearing impairments, diabetes, cancer, and dementias like Alzheimer's disease. Often, chronic conditions do not require the high-technology treatments offered in the health care system. Chronic conditions may be controlled with medication and regular contact with a physician or other health and social service professional. Persons with chronic conditions can continue to live at home or in the community, independently, with some help.

Unfortunately, the challenge of treating individuals with chronic conditions who also need assistance has been the increased costs of providing that care, especially if needed on a long-term basis. Factors that have contributed to these escalating costs are inflation, new technology, increasing institutional care costs, insurance risk, increasing regulation of service providers, and a growing population that needs the service. In addition, people believe that they have a right to any available health care treatment—no matter what the price. Programs like Medicare and Medicaid were founded on that premise: to guarantee access to health care for all who qualify. These public programs have continued to pay the bills for more and more expensive services for more and more people.

The health care delivery system has evolved with a focus on the medical, institutional model of care, because the cost of that was what was reimbursed. Social services, mental health services, and home health services fell outside of that narrow focus and have never received adequate public or private funding. As a result, providers structured services around what was reimbursable rather than what might have actually been needed. This fragmentation of supportive health services, in conjunction with medical services, challenges individuals with chronic conditions to try and manage their lives. Now, as we approach the 21st century, the combination of soaring health care costs and an expanding population in need is forcing a reexamination of the existing, fragmented, long-term care system.

While frail elderly and other dependent persons need affordable, long-term health and social services, public and private sectors try to control their expenditures without eliminating access for millions of individuals. This dilemma has caused much policy debate and service experimentation over the past 20 years. In this chapter, we examine projected population trends, and review public policy initiatives in long-term care that have been developed to reduce costs and to shore up a fragmented delivery system. Case management plays a major role in many of these solutions. Under appropriate circumstances, case management can help reduce some of the stress on an over-strained, long-term care system.

AGING IN AMERICA

Older persons have reaped the benefits of medical advancements by experiencing lower mortality rates with increased longevity. As the number of older adults living to age 65 years and beyond expands in proportion to the rest of the population, their influence, particularly on the health care system, also grows more powerful. Population projections indicate that from 1985 to 2020 persons aged 65 years and older will increase by 2% each year (that is approximately 750,000 persons per year), while the total United States population will increase by only 1% per year in that same time period (U.S. DHHS, 1987). The year 2020 will be a watershed one, because by then the post–World War II baby boom generation will have entered the ranks of the elderly. It is estimated that in 2020, the number of persons aged 65 years old will be double the number in 1985. That number is also a 50% increase in proportion to the general population: those persons 65 years and older will grow from 12% (in 1985) to 18% (in 2020) of the total population. This growth reflects nearly a 100% increase from 1970, when older adults represented 9.8% of the total population (Hollmann, 1989). The oldest-old, that is those persons living to age 85 and beyond, will double their proportion in the total population, growing from 1.2% to 2.4% during that period (U.S. DHHS, 1987). These population projections are conservative, based on the assumption that death rates will decrease at one-half the rate of decrease seen in 1980 and 1983. If this assumption is faulty and death rates continue to decline at the same rate, the numbers of the oldest-old, age 85 years and older, will be much greater (U.S. DHHS, 1987).

Older adults are a heterogeneous group, with an age span of

35 years (65 to 100 years old). In the oldest-old cohort, women make up almost 75% of the total. Predictions indicate that by 2020, the female-to-male ratio will be nearly one to one for those persons aged 65 to 74 years old. There will also be more elderly couples in the future. The minority population will also increase in proportion from 8% to 10% of the elderly. The older population prefers living in the southern or western states. It is estimated that during the 1990s the overall elderly population will increase by 20% in these areas, but the 85 years and older group will increase by 60%. Similarly, while the overall population will remain constant in the northeastern and north central states, the over 85 years old group is projected to expand by 33% (U.S.DHHS, 1987). As a whole, the elderly are not a wealthy group: average annual income for a household is around $15,000. They pay little in personal income taxes, such as Social Security or federal income taxes, but pay out a greater proportion of income on selective taxes, such as sales and interest-income taxes. The surprising, well-documented fact is that older adults outspend all other age groups on health care. The elderly pay between 17% and 27% of their budgets for health care (Estes, 1985).

Older adults are the primary users of health care services, whether it be a hospital or a nursing home, home health care, physician or dentist visits, or other services. Nearly 80% of them visit a doctor annually, 40% visit a dentist, 20% are hospitalized for short stays, 5% reside in nursing homes (U.S. DHHS, 1987; Population Reference Bureau, Inc., 1990), and approximately 4.4% use home health services of some kind (Berk & Bernstein, 1985). From the providers' perspective, however, older people compose the bulk of their clients. In 1980, approximately 25% of the oldest-old elderly were living in nursing homes but 40% of the nursing home residents were 85 years of age and older. By 2020, this oldest-old group will be 51% of the total nursing home population, and of this group it is predicted that nearly 20% will have Alzheimer's disease (Rivlin, Weiner, Henley, & Spence, 1988). For the nursing home employee, every other bed will be occupied by an 85-year-old person! The elderly are also the most intensive users of home health care. While they accounted for only 43% of the user population in 1979, the elderly received 77% of all home health care visits. By 2020, this user group is projected to nearly double in size, from 4.4% to 8%. At that time, almost 79% will be 75 years old or older (Rivlin et al., 1988; Palley & Oktay, 1989). These figures reflect purchased home health services only and do not include the many informal and family providers of home care. At current levels, the elderly account for 42% of hospital short-stay days, 20% of physicians' caseloads, 88% of nursing home beds, and 77% of home health visits. By 2020, they could increase their consumption to almost 50% of all hospital days, 25% of physician visits, and more than 90% of nursing home beds. Predictions of home health care use remain about the same. The potential utilization of services by older people could be nearly double the volume of 1980 by the year 2020. The implications for the health care system are awesome.

Despite these staggering predictions for increased utilization, it is still extremely difficult to ascertain which individuals will require which type of service, and what the costs will be for each person. Older persons coming of age in 2020 will be carrying with them the social and cultural effects of the latter part of the 20th century. By 2020, the elderly may be a better-educated group. Of those persons born between 1945 and 1949, 80% received their high school diploma, and 50% received some college education. They may be wealthier as a whole than their counterparts today. There will be a greater proportion of persons in the younger cohorts (age 65 years to 75 years) than today, as the baby boomers advance in age. By 2020, the elderly will have had greater exposure to health promotion and disease prevention. A good proportion will enjoy a healthier aging and maintain their productivity long past the present normal retirement age. Lastly, the elderly of 2020 will have experienced a lifelong connection with a service-oriented society that has been dealing with health care problems. They will be better prepared personally to face long-term care issues and better informed about how to take advantage of available services when health care needs arise (Cantor,

1991). Yet, while better informed and more willing to procure services for their health care needs, the 21st century consumers will still be unable to predict if a nursing home stay is in their future.

Many factors figure into the equation for the person most at risk of nursing home placement, which is considered to be the last and most expensive stop in the long-term care system. The most predictive factors are as follows: living alone, lack of available family supporters (especially a spouse), the number of limitations in the activities of daily living, mental impairment, and a recent hospital admission (Shapiro & Tate, 1988). The combination of two or more of these critical factors can lead to increasing utilization of formal health care services and contribute to the individual's health care expenditures. Figures from the United States Census Bureau on living arrangements for the elderly in 1989 demonstrate how older adults experience radical changes in their lives during their later years. At ages 65 years to 74 years, 63% of these older adults were married and living with their spouse, 25% lived alone, and 10% lived with other relatives. By age 85 years and older, only 4% lived with their spouse, 47% lived alone, and 28% lived with other relatives (Saluter, 1989). At this point in time, while our ability to predict the individual's future health care needs remains hazy, the present utilization rates give us insight into the aggregate needs of the future elderly population. We know with certainty that the full array of community health services offered, from hospital to nursing home to community to home, must be developed with an eye to providing access, managing cost, and assuring quality. All in all, the elderly are a major force influencing the health care delivery system today and will play a significant role in shaping the system to meet their needs of tomorrow.

PUBLIC POLICY TOWARD LONG-TERM CARE

Health care costs have been on the rise for the past 20 years, and, as stated previously, population projections point to more use of long-term care services at a greater expense to the consumer, the states, and the federal government. A growing awareness among these three groups is that few can afford these astronomical costs and that insurance coverage is often absent or inadequate. Nursing home residents may pay well over $40,000 per year for their care. Many private pay residents can expect to be come impoverished within their first year, and forced to apply for government assistance. The result is ever increasing pressure on the Medicaid program, which is designed to help the poor of any age gain access to health care, but which becomes by default the primary payor to nursing homes. Finding alternative, quality home care at a reasonable price can be extremely taxing for older persons with multiple, chronic conditions. Their family members are also confounded by the system as seen in the client example in Chapter 1. Few individuals have private insurance that covers the cost or range of services provided by the nursing and home care systems. Medicare pays for only a limited amount and specified type of nursing home and home health care and was never intended to cover long-term care, but rather was geared to insure individuals with acute, skilled care needs. When these acute episodes resolve, Medicare coverage ceases. For persons in need, financing home health care on a long-term basis can be a crushing expense. How did such a system evolve that is so complicated to arrange and expensive to pay for? A brief look at the public policy behind the health care delivery system and case management procedure evolved to meet long-term care needs is described in the remaining section of this chapter.

From 1930 to the 1960s, the premise underlying the federal outlay of funds for health care was simple; if the federal government invested enough money in the creation of basic health resources, such as hospitals, equipment, schools for training physicians and nurses, drug research, and others, then the necessary public services would be forthcoming. By the 1960s, however, it became obvious that no matter how massive the investment was, health problems were not being solved.

In 1965 the enactment of Title XVIII and Title XIX (Medicare and Medicaid) amendments to the Social Security Act radically changed the involvement of the federal government in health care by establishing a minimum level of health services for all poor and older people. Suddenly, all these older people and all the poor had guaranteed access to institutional health services and to a limited amount of home health care services. In contrast, the nonmedical, human service programs also expanded during the 1960s and early 1970s, but through restrictive, categorical funding that targeted specific needy groups such as crippled children, native Americans, veterans, the mentally ill, and others. Federal monies were stringently allocated to either medical or social service program categories, and this separation prevented individuals from achieving easy access to a full range of services.

In the late 1960s federal agencies did begin efforts toward encouraging a more cohesive system of health care. The Comprehensive Health Planning and Public Health Services Amendments of 1966 promoted the coordination of private and public sectors of health care. This partnership was intended to assist the development of regional and community health care systems (Kissick, 1970). At this time, case management began to surface as a method for helping individuals overcome the federal bureaucracy and improve their access to federal programs (Spitz & Abramson, 1987). Although it did not pass, the Allied Services Act of 1972 was introduced into Congress as a proposal to consolidate those social services utilizing case management to coordinate a full range of services. After 1965, when Medicare allocated limited funding for home health care, community-based home health care providers, once certified as eligible to participate in the Medicare program, could receive cost reimbursement for specified home health services. Medicare's narrow definition of home health care was limited to persons confined to their home, requiring part-time, intermittent, skilled nursing care, physical therapy, occupational therapy, or speech therapy. By 1966, however, fewer than 250 voluntary visiting nurse associations had the range of services necessary to meet the criteria set by Medicare for a home health agency.

It was not until the mid 1970s that legislation put significant dollars into the development of community resources for health care. In 1972, Section 222 of the Medicare Act authorized experiments in hospital and physician reimbursement, home care and day health services, and research and demonstration projects for community-based services. Many of these projects incorporated case management as a key service. Subsequently, in 1975, legislation enacted under Title XVIII of the Social Security Act and Titles III and V of the Older Americans Act funded home care services and other services such as meals, transportation, senior centers, and boarding facilities. By 1979, this infusion of public dollars into community services had resulted in approximately 3,000 home health care agencies becoming certified as Medicare providers (Quinn, 1986).

The 1980s saw continued development of community-based services through federal initiatives, but with a cost-conscious focus. For 15 years, the Medicare and Medicaid programs had far outpaced their original estimates for expenditures, and had added costs to the nation's climbing health care bill. The Omnibus Budget Reconciliation Act of 1980 broadened Medicare's reach into the home health care provider market through three critical changes. First, it loosened certification requirements for proprietary home health agencies and allowed these for-profit agencies to become certified even in states without licensing laws. Second, the act eliminated the three-day prior hospitalization requirement for coverage of home health services in Medicare Part A. And finally, it eliminated the 100-visit limitation of coverage in Part A. As a result, the private home health care industry boomed. Between 1982 and 1984, the number of proprietary home health agencies expanded by 300%, representing 30% of all home health agencies (Palley & Oktay, 1989).

In the Omnibus Budget Reconciliation Act of 1981, an attempt was made to reform the Medicaid program by allowing states to modify Medicaid regulations. Section 2176 of this act designated a "waiver mechanism" that allowed states to implement projects that provided a significant number of community-based health and social services to clients with similar needs through a central funding source, as well as compensate the clients for services not otherwise available. The state could apply for three "waivers" that either limited the service offered from being a statewide program (Medicaid regulations stated that the program benefits must be offered to all state residents), allowed reimbursement for services not ordinarily part of the state's Medicaid plan, or allowed for modification of the existing eligibility criteria for the client applying to the Medicaid program. The importance of this policy change was that a public program could now include a range of both health- and personal-care services and case management services through one funding source. A drawback was that these services were tied to a means-test for eligibility.

The federal government gave states room to experiment; at the same time, it clearly intended to find ways to reduce growing Medicaid costs. The traditional Medicaid approach to health care was through a welfare system, with eligibility based on a means-test. This was different from the Medicare program in which eligibility is determined by age and disability. By its design, Medicaid filled in the gaps where the private sector was absent and where the Medicare program was inadequate. These factors contributed to the unforeseen expenses of the Medicaid program (Stevens & Stevens, 1970). As part of the same Omnibus Budget Reconciliation Act of 1981, the federal government announced the reduction of federal matching payments to each state for the Medicaid program, encouraging the states to look for money-saving programs with their new freedoms. In response, many states focused their efforts on reducing costs incurred by older people, who were the most intensive users of expensive nursing home and hospital care. States developed programs that screened nursing home applicants before admission and offered community-based service alternatives instead of institutionalization. These new programs had the ability to integrate health and social services for clients of all ages, and, in effect, were capable of handling persons with chronic care needs. By 1986 the Health Care Financing Administration had approved 104 waivers from 41 states. Case management was offered as a Medicaid reimbursed service in 85% of the states with programs (Applebaum & Austin, 1990; Palley & Oktay, 1989).

As the states developed their Medicaid waiver programs, the federal government initiated a national experiment in community-based, long-term care for the elderly. Starting in 1980, 10 sites were chosen across the country to implement the National Long-Term Care Channeling Demonstration. This demonstration was designed to test a comprehensive case management approach through two different models. Both models, the basic and the financial control, channeled services to clients through a central point of intake, assessment, and on-going case management. The targeted clients were the severely impaired elderly who required long-term care services for an extended period, and who were at risk of entering a nursing home. From 1982 to 1985, the demonstration tested two types of managed care, five of each, in ten sites. In the Basic Model, case managers coordinated available community services for clients and had authority over a small amount of service funds, like Title III and Social Service Block Grant monies. In the Financial Model, the case managers had authority over pooled funds (waivered Medicaid and Medicare dollars) that could be used to pay for a full range of services. Through these two approaches, case managers attempted to use community services, both formal and informal, in lieu of institutional care whenever possible and appropriate. The Channeling demonstration sought to improve the quality of life for severely impaired elderly while simultaneously reducing the cost of long-term care for these individuals. After its conclusion, the Channeling demonstration had a positive influence on newly implemented statewide case management programs, as many Channeling staff played significant roles in program development and operation in the Medicaid case management programs. Several states adopted the Channeling assessment instrument for their case management programs. Eight of the ten original demonstrations are still operating, through different funding mechanisms (Carcagno et al., 1986).

Another current demonstration, begun under the auspices of the Deficit Reduction Act of 1984, is the Social/Health Maintenance Organization (S/HMO). This project started operations in 1985 under the guidance of Brandeis University at four sites across the country. The S/HMO design is a consolidation of services and providers, similar to an HMO, but includes the full range of services from acute medical and supplemental health to case management services for chronic care. Chronic care services include homemaker, personal care, respite care, adult day health care, transportation, and others. The S/HMO design also involves the consolidation of financing. By pooling all funding, such as Medicare, Medicaid, private premiums, and client cost sharing, the S/HMO avoids the regulatory and reimbursement constraints of the current system. Individuals enroll in the organization and pay premiums as members to receive services. Enrollees, then, should represent ideally the whole spectrum of elderly persons, including healthy and frail. In this model, the burden is upon the case manager to manage service dollars judiciously because payments for services are capitated and prospective. Because providers are prepaid a fixed amount for their services, even nursing home care is covered up to a certain amount. The S/HMO has a strong incentive to contain its costs for each client. If the cost for providing services to enrollees exceeds revenues, the S/HMO suffers the financial loss. One goal of the S/ HMO is to ascertain whether case management can control the cost of in-home and community services for members through the efficient use of resources, balancing the expensive with the less expensive services, while providing the best care possible (Applebaum & Austin, 1990; Greenberg & Levitz, 1984).

In spite of the availability of federal and state funding and expanded community services, the client still derives little benefit from the total system. Because these services are implemented by policy and not by client demand, the individual is likely to find that the services available may not fit her needs or that she is not eligible for the services even if in need. Through the research and demonstration projects funded by Medicare and Medicaid waivers, new methods of dealing with a fragmented delivery system and the complicated health care needs of the chronically impaired are being continually explored. Case management is one promising means for linking together the provider system, coordinating funding sources, and screening users of services to determine the most appropriate level of care to meet their needs.

LESSONS LEARNED FROM THE DEMONSTRATIONS

Publicly financed demonstration projects have spanned over a decade of experimentation, beginning between 1970 and 1985. They have explored creative solutions to problems of health, financing care, services, reimbursement, quality of care, access and equality of care, and specific types of care needed by individuals with long-term, chronic care needs.

The fundamental hypothesis tested by these projects was whether community care could be a cost-effective substitute for institutional care. It is well documented that, given the choice, individuals would prefer to remain at home rather than enter an institution. One key goal of the projects was to identify those individuals at risk of institutionalization by developing specific eligibility criteria to determine levels of frailty. Through this method, these identified individuals might either avoid or delay entering a nursing home by using extensive community-based services (Kemper, Applebaum, & Harrigan, 1987).

The long-term care projects employed three primary strategies for reform: first, to develop, coordinate, and upgrade the long-term care delivery system (Triage, Georgia Alternative Health Services, New York's Nursing Home Without Walls, and others); second, to control client access to and utilization of institutional services (ACCESS, South Carolina Long-Term Care Project); and third, to consolidate long-term care services delivery into a single agency (On Lok, Social/Health Maintenance Organizations) (Applebaum & Austin, 1990).

The demonstration projects also experimented with differing case management models for long-term care as a means to develop plans of care and deliver services. The determination of the model was dependent on the type of financing available in each demonstration. Three separate models at work throughout the projects are described as follows.

The *Broker Model* is the simplest design for case management. Case managers act as brokers for clients and service providers by linking up the two through a referral system. Case managers have no service dollars to spend on the client's behalf; hence, no means for guaranteeing that services are indeed delivered as prescribed. This particular model functions well in a community rich in services, because the client has many provider options to choose from and the case manager has no direct conflict of interest with the various providers. Many of the demonstrations (e.g., the Basic Channeling projects) used this model in part, because few had complete control over service funds and had to refer clients to existing services, but none were based exclusively on the broker concept. The major drawback to the broker system, and the reason demonstrations did not rely solely on it, is that the broker can only coordinate the existing service providers and does not effect any real change or develop new services in the overall delivery system.

The *Service Management Model* is the most commonly used design in the demonstrations. In this model, case managers do have funds available for services, but are restricted by a cost cap on care plans, usually 60% to 80% of a comparable nursing home stay. Since many of the projects took advantage of the Medicaid and Medicare waivers, case managers could authorize a full range of services for clients without the usual funding constraints connected with traditional public programs. A good example of this model is illustrated in the 2176 (Medicaid) waiver programs, many of which are nursing home preadmission screening projects. Once the client meets the initial eligibility requirements for Medicaid and shows functional deficits, the case manager has the authority to allocate the monies for services not usually covered under the Medicaid plan according to the needs of the client.

The *Managed Care Model* builds on the previous two models with one new twist, prospective financing. Case managers have control over a pool of funds, similar to the Service Management Model, to purchase services for clients; however, providers are prepaid a specific amount, placing the liability on them for excess costs. In this process, the case managers play a crucial role in allocating limited resources to a careful, efficient plan of care. The On Lok demonstration was the first project to operate under this managed care system, and its results fostered the development of the S/HMO. The S/HMO, because its members are enrollees, is itself at risk for any cost overruns in services rendered.

These demonstrations developed, in one form or another, means for integrating both fragmented funding sources and diverse health and social services. By doing so, they attempted to improve the continuity and quality of care for the individual and simultaneously create cost-effective methods for the delivery of long-term care services. Yet, the expanded development and use of community services for this frail population raised several concerns. First of all, if the government extended its reimbursement (through the waiver mechanism) to more community-based services, this effort might encourage more users to "come out of the woodwork" and push up overall costs. This increase in community-based users could, in turn, outweigh any savings accrued from reduced nursing home use. Second, the availability of these new formal services could supplant the existing informal support services, and, therefore, add more costs to the government health care bill (Greenberg and Levitz, 1984; Rivlin et al., 1988).

The demonstrations provided answers to both of these concerns, as well as raising even more issues. The demonstration project experiences revealed the feasibility of substituting community-based services for nursing home care for certain individuals. The South Carolina Long-Term Care project was a good example of how expanded community services in combination with preadmission nursing home screening can reduce overall nursing home use. Also, as earlier stated, many of the demonstrations incorporated cost limits for community services per individual at 60% to 85% of nursing home reimbursement rates. The Financial Channeling project implemented a cap on expenditures for its total caseload, but average expenses fell below 60% of the nursing home rate. Several projects developed cost sharing plans with clients, in which clients with higher incomes paid a share of their service costs. When drawing a cost comparison, however, the advantage of community care over nursing home care diminishes as a client's needs for services increase. Yet, in terms of reducing the rate of placement in a nursing home, the demonstration data showed no significant reduction overall. This result pointed out that by expanding community-based programs other needy individuals are identified, beyond those at risk, who could benefit from home care services. While costs for certain individuals may indeed be less when community services are utilized, the aggregate program costs may actually rise over time (Kemper et al., 1987).

The demonstrations also attempted to develop targeting criteria that would measure client frailty to identify those most at risk of nursing home placement. Most projects defined frailty through a combination of age, functional need, and service need. Some demonstrations served only the elderly with a minimum age of 50 to 65 years. Others served the adult disabled, while one served clients of any age. Several projects mapped out specific disability requirements for eligibility; for example, the Channeling project defined functional impairment as two limitations in the Activities of Daily Living Scale (ADL), or three limitations in the Instrumental Activities of Daily Living Scale (IADL). Other projects required service needs to qualify for enrollment; for example, the New York City Home Care Project defined at-risk clients as those needing help with personal care for eight to 20 hours per week. A few projects deemed clients eligible if they met the Medicaid requirements for admission to a nursing home. Some projects combined two areas of frailty: the Channeling demonstration criteria also accepted individuals with one ADL and two IADLs, and who needed help in two or more service categories for six months or more or who had a fragile informal support system. The demonstrations found that client frailty did increase in conjunction with the exactness of the disability requirements.

As a means to develop, coordinate, and upgrade the long-term care system, the projects took advantage of the waivers in Medicaid and Medicare to expand community services and extend authorization power of case managers. Case managers could use expanded services to reach more individuals for a longer time than programs normally allowed. For example, projects extended in-home services to cover nonhealth services such as homemaking, personal care, chore services, home-delivered meals, and companion services; and they extended coverage to additional community services such as adult day care, foster care, medical equipment, mental health counseling, and respite care. By extending the case manager's authorization power for services, the projects allowed the case manager to order Medicare reimbursed home health aide services or social services financed by Social Service block grant funds when the need arose. The case manager could at last manage a client's services instead of being just a broker or an advocate on the client's behalf. The demonstrations also refuted the contention that expanded formal services would reduce the participation of the informal support system in long-term care. In fact, although caregivers did take advantage of the services available, their caretaking abilities were reinforced through the formal supports, allowing them to continue assistance for a longer period of time.

Controlling access to nursing homes was another strategy used in an effort to manage costs. Two demonstrations focused primarily on this endeavor, and one, the South Carolina Long-Term Care Project, showed the most positive results. Both ACCESS and the South Carolina project were designed as pre-admission screening programs for nursing homes. Each could withhold authorization for nursing home payment if, after review, the individual did not meet eligibility criteria. The South Carolina project showed that with case managers screening all the clients, nursing home use was reduced by 31% per year (Kemper et al., 1987). These results identified a high-risk population who met the Medicaid criteria for admission before they entered a nursing home. As noted earlier, many states have implemented similar programs, based on the findings of these particular demonstrations, in hopes of predicting with greater accuracy who will need the services of a nursing home and who can remain in the community.

Currently, two projects are exploring the possibilities of consolidation of long-term care services into a single organization. The On Lok project has even incorporated acute medical services to accommodate the fullest range of services imaginable for a select group of clients: it includes physician care, hospital services, and nursing home care. No other projects covered these acute medical services, except the Triage, Inc., project in the mid 1970s. The S/HMO follows its predecessor by integrating the acute and chronic care services into one system and by consolidating all levels of the long-term care system: provider, population, finance, and risk (Kemper et al., 1987). Physicians work together with chronic care case managers in the program. The On Lok Replication Projects are continuing to test this model of service delivery. The S/HMO projects are still in the mid-level stages of development. The goal is to attract enough members to make the S/HMO a viable alternative for the elderly population.

While the demonstrations documented no significant reduction in costs, they did show evidence of increased benefits to the persons receiving care. Measuring life quality in quantitative terms is impossible; yet, if individuals are more content with expanded community services, perhaps the benefits to society outweigh the costs. As Kemper et al. (1987) state, "The contribution of the community care demonstrations should be to move the research and policy debate beyond the question of whether expanded public financing of community care will reduce costs to how much community care society is willing to pay for, who should receive it, and how it can be delivered efficiently." Case management has great potential for improving the efficiency and effectiveness of the delivery system.

Finally, it is important to give new and existing programs the flexibility to change how they operate, based on their experience, and to investigate alternative ways to meet the needs of clients, reimbursers, and providers in the care system. Experimentation should be encouraged as we strive to create an accessible, equitable, and affordable long-term care system.

Assessment

3

> Each person is unique with specific needs, goals and preferences. Individuals have a right to autonomy, to make their own decisions, and to exercise control over their own lives. Case management maximizes the capacity of the individual and his or her caregiver to make informed and appropriate decisions in arranging for needed care. (Connecticut Community Care, Inc., Case Management Institute, on the Philosophy of Case Management, 1990)

REFERRAL AND PRESCREENING

The Organizational Setting

The versatility of case management enables it to adapt to a range of existing service delivery mechanisms. Case management programs may be part of a variety of organizational settings and their program goals defined by the populations that they serve. Current organizations that may employ case management services include family service agencies, area agencies on aging, hospitals, municipal health departments, health maintenance organizations, social/health maintenance organizations, mental health and developmentally disabled groups, insurance companies, free-standing case management entities, government human service departments, and home health agencies. Funds for case management and other services may come from public and private resources, such as federal, state, and county dollars, and foundation and philanthropic grants, insurers, and private individuals. Many agencies offer individuals components of the case management function, such as initial limited evaluation and referral, consultation services, and assessment services.

If the program is reimbursed using public funds or insurance payments, eligibility requirements for the program are established by the payor. For example, a program funded with state monies may determine that all clients must meet the state's Medicaid eligibility requirements before receiving case management services. Private payors, like insurance companies, may impose certain functional disability levels, preexisting conditions, and other requirements that clients must meet to qualify for services. A free-standing agency that receives funds from both public and private sources usually maintains several separate caseloads of clients accepted under different eligibility rules. In contrast, a fee-for-service client, unfettered by funding restraints, does not have to meet income or functional status requirements to be the recipient of case management services.

The level of case management delivered may vary from simple referral only to comprehensive services, and may involve short- or long-term client contact. For instance, a hospital-based program with discharge planner case managers may be concerned only with making the patient's discharge and transition back home a smooth one. After setting up a care plan for the client and monitoring the client's recuperation for a limited period, this discharge planner case manager would have completed the institutional mission. For a long-term care insurance policy beneficiary, the approach would be far different. The case manager in this example would be concerned with the client's acute and chronic care needs for as long as necessary, within limits covered in the specific policy. In a fee for service program, the client would dictate the terms of the client/case management relationship. The client may opt to purchase only consultation services from the agency, or the client may choose to purchase a larger package of services, such as assessment, and ongoing case management for as long as necessary. Comprehensive case management services could be unbundled into separate, component parts, and the client would determine the level and duration of services desired.

The Referral Process

With program goals and eligibility requirements in place, the case management agency will most likely begin to target potential clients. Eligibility requirements will define most of the criteria for determining the client population. For instance, many programs have age limits, serving individuals between the ages of 18 and 65 years, or just adults over 65 years old, or only children under 18 years old, or specific groups (the mentally retarded, traumatic brain injured people, etc.). Most programs also require pre-determined levels of client frailty to qualify for case management services, such as requiring the client to have deficits in two Activities of Daily Living (ADLs) or a combination of deficits in Instrumental Activities of Daily Living (IADLs), ADLs, and cognitive disability. (Most of the later, post-1980, demonstration projects discussed in Chapter 2 based eligibility on these functional incapacities.) Geographic boundaries are another method used to target clients for a program. Certain funding sources have attached restrictions on where monies can be spent, within city, county, and regional limits. Programs also impose restrictions on allowable income; most publicly-funded programs intend to serve the poor and frail who would otherwise not be financially able to find assistance. Old age, poverty, and functional disabilities tend to be key factors included in most public programs. By design, these programs handle the most frail and the most expensive clients, those who are the heaviest users of the broadest range of long-term care services, including case management. For these programs, the difficulty is trying to maintain a case mix that offsets the expensive end of the caseload. Individuals with

IADL deficiencies, such as the inability to shop, wash laundry, and cook, may be less expensive to support than those with several ADL deficiencies, such as the inability to bathe, dress, and transfer. In fact, the number of older adult clients with multiple ADL deficits is increasing. The Urban Institute forecasts that by the year 2030 nearly 14 million persons age 65 years and older will need help with one or more ADLs. This increase is over twice the number (6.2 million) of persons requiring this type of help in 1990 (Lawlor, 1990). Presently, 47% of the elderly aged 85 years and older live alone. With the growth in the number of individuals in this oldest-old age bracket (3.3% annually) combined with the fact that nearly 50% will likely live alone, more persons with ADLs and personal care needs will be looking to community services for assistance (Saluter, 1989). Fee-for-service clients will continue to grow in number. Individuals with resources can have the services they need as long as those resources last. However, it is just as important for the case manager to help the private-pay individuals plan and conserve their resources for as long as possible by judiciously planning for appropriate services.

Having clearly identified the target population, the program's next step is to locate clients. Several means for identifying potential clients are:

- Introducing your program to community agencies and familiarizing them with the type of clients you can serve. These agencies can then refer potential clients, that they come into contact with, to your agency.
- Referrals from your own clients, and from their families, who know others in the community that could benefit from the program.
- Community outreach by case managers and case management administrators to: civic and church groups, news agencies, newspapers, senior centers and organizations, employee assistance programs of local companies, chapters of professional organizations, and others.
- Marketing efforts to the community through: brochures, advertising, business bureaus, chambers of commerce, and contact with private organizations.

The Prescreening Process

Just as all companies screen incoming calls, each case management program must institute some system for initial contact with clients. The prescreening process determines the likelihood of a client needing case management services by identifying those who meet established eligibility criteria and who need a full assessment. As a prelude to entry into the case management system, the prescreening step eliminates inappropriate client assessments, saves valuable case manager and client time, and conserves agency resources.

Program goals and eligibility requirements define the prescreening process. With the variety of case management programs in existence, each may determine eligibility using different criteria. Regardless of the type of program, the prescreening process should include several fundamental elements as a means to identify appropriate clients. The National Council on Aging, through its affiliate the National Institute of Community-Based Long-Term Care, has developed a set of Care Management Standards. These standards include the general elements recommended for a thorough prescreening of individuals. They are as follows:

- obtain background information, such as name, age, marital status, living arrangement;
- determine reason for the referral or for the individual's seeking help;
- determine what supports are already available (informal and formal);
- evaluate the need for immediate action (e.g., crisis intervention, protective services);
- determine eligibility of the applicant in relation to income, age, or other requirements; and/or,
- determine sufficient need to warrant assessment. (National Institute on Community-based Long-Term Care, 1988)

One additional element that should be established at the prescreening stage if possible, is the client's or caregiver's interest in the program and desire for services offered, especially if referred by a provider agency. The case manager assesses client and caregiver, identifies problems, and seeks solutions that benefit both parties. In turn, both parties must be active participants in the process, supplying information, discussing their problems, and participating in establishing preliminary goals. Clients who do not wish to participate in this process and caregivers who manifest a lukewarm attitude as supporters of the client may not want to be involved with a case management program, which is their right. They may be more comfortable purchasing services on their own. A thorough prescreening procedure should be able to detect such nuances by asking the right questions at the outset, saving both time and money.

Upon referral to the case management agency, Evelyn was very depressed and not meeting the expectations of her physical and occupational therapists. She had multiple functional difficulties subsequent to a pulmonary embolism and a stroke. She lived with her daughter and three preschool-age grandchildren.

When the telephone interview began, Evelyn was quiet and subdued. As the interview progressed, however, she grew more animated and articulate about her depression and living situation. Evelyn explained that being home bound had increased her feelings of isolation. She described the strained relationship between her daughter and herself, primarily due to the reversal of their traditional roles. She expressed her anger and frustration at being physically incapacitated and functionally limited. After the case manager spoke about working on these problems with Evelyn, she understood the case management role and was eager to use case management services to ameliorate her situation (Connecticut Community Care, Inc., 1985).

Successful prescreening can improve the cost effectiveness of a case management program by minimizing the amount of case manager time spent on inappropriate referrals or assessments, and it can reduce consumer confusion and wasted time by referring the client to the most suitable resources for her needs. This first level of case management function is extremely important for a significant number of older and disabled adults and their families who face the conundrum of long-term care for the very first time. A good example of prescreening at work on a large scale is the previously mentioned nursing home preadmission screening program, funded through state Medicaid programs under a federal waiver and subcontracted to case management organizations. Designed to reduce inappropriate placement in a nursing home, these programs identify clients who still can handle independent living and, with help, remain in or return to the community.

Sophie had dependencies in all IADLs and most ADLs. She transferred and walked poorly. She lived in a walk-up apartment and could not climb the stairs by herself. Her sister was living with her temporarily, and the two women bickered constantly. After screening by a case manager, Sophie was placed immediately in a nursing home, due to her low functional ability and safety issues at home. The case manager maintained contact with Sophie while she lived in the nursing home to determine if she might be able to return to the community. After seven months of rehabilitation therapy in the nursing home, the case manager helped Sophie locate an apartment modified for the handicapped in a senior citizens complex. The case manager and Sophie then worked out a care plan for her new living situation that included family support, money management, home health aide services, and on-going case management services (Connecticut Community Care, Inc., 1985).

Methods of Prescreening

The prescreening process can be the first contact between a client and the case management agency. The foremost concern at this stage is to ensure each potential client equal access to case management services. The prescreening interview is composed of uniform, universally applicable questions. These carefully designed questions try to elicit accurate information from clients and supporters regarding the client's situation. Studies have found prescreens to be approximately 80% accurate in the information gathered, with the errors attributed to the client's underreporting of a problem. For this interview, the questions are compiled in a prescreening instrument which can later provide a transition to the assessment. Many programs may design a prescreening tool for automated data entry, further facilitating the flow of information from prescreen to assessment.

A number of questions may be raised by the prescreening process. Where is the prescreen performed? Is it done by another agency which sends the information along to the case management program, or is it performed in-house? Is it completed on the telephone or in-person? A telephone interview is obviously the least costly method for prescreening; however, information gathered on the telephone can differ from that gathered in the home. In the home, the case manager can observe the client's environment and functional capabilities firsthand and instantly verify many of the client's statements about her condition and needs. The most accurate method for prescreening is to conduct the interview with the client in-person; however, most case management organizations cannot afford to perform the prescreen in this manner. Considering the high degree of accuracy linked with the telephone prescreen, many agencies prefer to use the telephone first and follow-up with an assessment visit. The case manager can then reconfirm prescreening information face-to-face with the client, ideally in the client's home environment.

Who performs the prescreen? Wherever the prescreen is performed, the staff involved must be specially trained for the task. The personnel do not need to be case managers. Support staff, such as case manager assistants, and other administrative support personnel can be taught to do thorough and consistent prescreenings. In the National Channeling Demonstration, paraprofessionals were responsible for prescreening applicants. The demonstration viewed this step as the least professionalized of the case management functions (Capitman, Haskins, & Berstein, 1986). However, if staff lack the proper preparation and training needed to conduct a prescreen, the value of a prescreen is jeopardized. Formal training for prescreeners should include the following:

Telephone etiquette: How to ask questions of a personal nature. How to ask questions in a logical sequence: What is the problem? How long have you had it? What do you think about it? What have you done about it?

Communication skills: Basic interviewing skills, such as listening skills; sensitivity to and awareness of ethnic and cultural differences; techniques for drawing out information from clients

Handling difficult situations: A client grows angry during the interview, or becomes upset or seems depressed; a client refuses to answer questions or gives bizarre responses

Instruction on how to use the prescreening instrument: Practice interviews, proper documentation methods (some agencies might enter information directly into a computer file, requiring staff to learn data entry techniques)

Use of personal judgement during the interview: When to consult with the supervisor or case managers. Prescreening personnel must rely heavily on the clinical judgement of supervisors or more experienced case managers regarding difficult cases and must be comfortable consulting with other staff, as necessary. (Connecticut Community Care, Inc., 1991)

The prescreening process acts as a gatekeeper to the agency's programs. The variety of possible public and private case management programs discussed earlier all carry inherent constraints as to the type and number of clients enrolled. During the prescreening process, clients are evaluated according to program criteria to determine eligibility for particular programs. After acceptance via the prescreen, the client will move directly to the next phase, assessment. Most programs establish an allowable time frame between the two stages, perhaps seven days or two weeks as in the Channeling Demonstration, but this allotted time may also be modified to reflect the severity and immediacy of client needs. Those clients with immediate needs may move more quickly through the two stages than those with less immediate needs. Programs must develop a method for prioritizing clients through the prescreening mechanism. The high priority situations should be clearly defined by program administration for the personnel involved in prescreening potential clients.

The capacity of the case management program to enroll new clients is another factor which influences the prescreening process. Some programs, like many mandatory nursing home preadmission screening programs, are financed through entitlement funds; everyone applying to a nursing home, who is eligible for Medicaid, must be screened prior to admission. Those who are deemed appropriate for a nursing home level of care may be referred to the case management agency for arrangement of alternative services in a community setting, if possible. These individuals will be supported by Medicaid funds because of their entitlement status, and the case management agency will be paid for services rendered to the clients. If the case management program is operating under a discretionary program which limits both the dollars available for services and the number of clients that can be served, prescreening may take on a different role. For instance, if the caseload is at capacity, applicants who are prescreened and meet eligibility criteria must be placed on a waiting list until a vacancy opens for program services.

The waiting list can create a different set of problems for the organization: How is it handled and by whom? The waiting list should be handled under the same eligibility guidelines as the case management program itself. The existence of a waiting list underscores the importance of accurate prescreening. What client would react happily to being told, after waiting one month for services, that upon review she is not and was not eligible for the case management program. The clients on the waiting list must be reevaluated by some protocol when service becomes available. Two options are likely:

Chronological: Clients are taken off of the waiting list in the same order they were put on; first come, first served.

Prioritization: While the first option is simple enough, it does not take into account those clients with severe, immediate needs. Prioritizing through a needs analysis may be a more equitable method in certain case management programs—again depending on program goals and constraints. Priority status could be determined by age, available support system, health status, environmental problems, financial resources, and functional deficits. By using a rating scale for each factor and the clinical judgement of the case manager, a combination high score of need could be determined.

An alternative for the agency is to offer case management on a fee-for-service basis to waiting-list clients. Clients may be able to afford some needed services through private means, and select this option as a temporary solution. When a program vacancy appears, the client could transfer into the appropriate program.

COMPREHENSIVE ASSESSMENT

Once prescreening is completed and the client is eligible for case management service, an assessment is scheduled. The information gathered at time of assessment is determined by the requirements of the programs that the case management agency is administering. The assessment may be as brief as eligibility determination—asking questions focused on age, sex, specific disability criteria, income, and assets. This level of case management may be used by county and city social service departments. At the other end of the spectrum is comprehensive assessment, a multi-dimensional process that provides a detailed profile of the client's needs and resources. Case management programs using this comprehensive assessment would most likely serve clients with multiple, chronic disabilities requiring a variety of services over a long period of time. Case managers involved in this type of assessment must be well-educated as clinicians and very knowledgeable about long-term care services in the community. For the purposes of this book, the comprehensive assessment model is presented.

Client assessment is the foundation on which case management stands. The gathering and analysis of comprehensive assessment data results in the client being served in a most effective and efficient manner. For clients with multiple, chronic care needs, the assessment gathers information from all areas in order to holistically evaluate each client's unique situation. The goal of the assessment process is to systematically organize client data into a manageable form, and provide a basis for the analysis and identification of the strengths and weaknesses of the client and the caregivers. With this firm base in place, the case manager can then build a care plan that supports the strengths, compensates for the weaknesses, and restores as healthful a balance as possible to the client's life.

Comprehensive client assessment includes data from each of the seven domains mentioned in Chapter 1: health, emotional/behavioral status, cognitive ability, functional level, support system, environment, and finances. The assessment can be a time-consuming process, but well worth the effort; because, if client problems are not adequately identified at the onset, the case manager cannot develop effective solutions. For instance, a case manager thinks that a client should move into housing for the handicapped, because she can no longer climb the stairs to her apartment, and she is too far away from the market to walk and carry groceries back home. After questioning her further, however, the case manager finds that the client has lived most of her life in this neighborhood, feels safe, and has friends nearby. While the new apartment would be more suitable for the client's functional capabilities, the new surroundings could cause enormous emotional stress for the client, which would far outweigh the more functional living accommodations. The case manager, cognizant of the client's feelings and values, might decide to provide more assistance to the client in her present surroundings and avoid the anxiety tied to moving. The case manager's goal during assessment is to identify problems the client is having in any of the seven domains mentioned previously. The questions are designed to identify the client's ability to function or manage in each area and then focus on specific strengths and problems within each area. These questions are carefully arranged in the assessment instrument. While there are a number of assessment instruments in use, each should have the following characteristics:

- facilitate the collection of clinically relevant information;
- provide a basis for the justification of the plan of care; and,
- incorporate objective measures that enable clients to be compared over time and across care settings. (Kane & Kane, 1991)

Commonly, the assessment tool must serve the dual purposes of case management clinical practice and programmatic requirements, such as, program eligibility, reporting requirements, and research. This can present real challenges in instrument development. Instrument design should meet the following criteria.

First, the instrument needs to be acceptable to both the client and the case manager, by providing an appropriate framework for the assessment interview. The client must feel comfortable responding to questions. If certain questions seem too invasive, the client should have the option of not answering them. The case manager must be familiar with the instrument questions and at ease with the format, thus allowing the questions to flow smoothly and in a sensible, logical order. Insensitive questioning is upsetting to clients and might even damage the future relationship between the client and case manager. Rapport and trust between the client and case manager begin at the time of initial assessment and are crucial in developing an ongoing relationship. The assessment instrument, logically structured, provides for the exchange of information in a sequential manner.

Second, the assessment should be completed within a reasonable amount of time. In the Channeling Demonstration, case managers regularly reported that the instrument was too long, considering the length of time to complete it, the associated paperwork, and the burden to the client (Carcagno et al., 1986). The initial assessment interview can consume, at a minimum, two to three hours of case manager time. This does not include staff time, following the interview, doing telephone work to corroborate assessment information and speaking with supporters and others involved with the client, and used in data entry (for programs with automated client assessment systems) and clerical procedures. The time invested in completing a thorough, comprehensive assessment, however, will reward the case manager later through knowledge and efficiency in managing the on-going care plan. The key is to find or develop an instrument that is comprehensive, yet supplies a basic approach to information without unnecessary questions.

Third, the assessment instrument must meet the multiple informational needs of the case management organization and its contractors. Client assessment data become the basis for determining case manager clinical accountability and assure quality of the service provided by the agency. Supervisory staff should be able to review a client's care plan, the baseline assessment information, and the case manager's clinical notes, and understand the clinical reasoning used to formulate the care plan. The information should be easily accessible for review and for comparison with later reassessment information and care plan changes. The agency must routinely evaluate the quality of its case management services by reviewing the quality of client assessment and reassessment data, clinical notes, and all other relevant information. Problems identified during assessment should be properly addressed in the care plan.

Fourth, assessment instruments utilize measurement scales that have been determined to be valid and reliable. All sections of the assessment instrument are completed. Common assessment domains are described under the following areas.

Health: Health-related information provides the case manager with an overview of the client's physical stability, and, in some situations, of new or unevaluated symptoms for which the client needs to be referred for further evaluation. Health evaluation includes past and present history of illness and hospitalization, a review of current symptoms, a listing of current medications, and ratings of sensory capabilities such as hearing and vision, of communication skills, and of the client's self-perception of health. Client perception of health status is a good starting point in gathering health information, because of the insight this provides into the health issues the client considers to be most significant. Sources of data include: hospital records or community referral; objective observation by the case manager regarding the client's capabilities, including hearing/vision; or, a modified physical examination completed by the nurse case manager or released from the client's physician.

Emotional Status: In the emotional/behavioral domain, the case manager has the opportunity to evaluate the client's mood/affect and determine the presence of troublesome behaviors. The client's emotional outlook and coping style is revealed in responses to direct questions concerning emotional status. The client's feelings, social functioning, and behavior are included in this area of questioning. The measurement of social stress in the client's life is important. Death of a spouse, retirement, relocation, major illness, and death of a friend or a pet are important considerations when evaluating a client's emotional status. The "Measurement of Functional Activities in Older Adults in the Community" (Pfeffer & Kurosaki, 1982) is designed as an index of social function to identify areas where assistance is needed and whether cognitive and affective (mood) changes signify social dysfunction. Performance in everyday life is often linked more directly to social independence than to test results. Some clients continue to attend church, clubs, and other events in the face of situations that alone might indicate a frail, dependent person.

Cognitive Ability: The cognitive tests are of a screening nature, capturing some measure of the client's memory and practical judgement at a point in time. The presence of troublesome behavior may be related to cognitive functioning and can have a significant influence on the client's ability to remain in the community. This domain assesses the client's mental status through specific tasks that may include measures of the client's orientation, attention, construction, calculation, recent and remote memory, and the ability to reason and make judgements. The "Mental Status Questionnaire" (MSQ), developed by Kahn and Goldfarb in 1960, consists of 10 memory questions focussing on orientation and memory. Sample questions are: What is today's date? What is your address? How old are you? Who is president? Who was the previous president? Other measures of cognitive function are: "Short Portable Mental Status Questionnaire (SPMSQ)" (Pfeiffer, 1975), "Folstein Mini-Mental Status Exam" (Folstein, Folstein, & McHugh, 1975), "Cognitive Capacity Screen" (Jacobs, Bernard, Delgado, Strain, 1977), and the "Set Test" (Isaac & Kennie, 1973). In this last test, the client names as many items as possible in four sets: fruits, animals, colors, and towns, up to 10 items. Fifteen out of 40 indicates abnormality. This is a good test for differentiating demented from non-demented populations. Another test that evaluates the presence of affective disorders, especially depression, is the "Zung Self-Rating Depression Scale" (Zung, 1965). For the case manager, the client's cognitive ability is an important factor in determining whether the client is capable, safe, and able to manage in the community. The case manager must be careful not to view the client separately from the support network of family and friends. The information gathered from cognitive measurements must be interpreted in conjunction with information about client supporters before deciding upon appropriate intervention methods. A severely cognitively impaired client who lives with a spouse may only require respite services (for the spouse), while the same individual living alone might require much more intensive services.

Functional Level: Functional assessment scales are crucial to the care planning process because they identify the client's ability to perform personal care and household management tasks. Information generated in this area can help case managers identify what services will be needed by the individual to stay in the present environment, and also what level of care (e.g. intermediate or skilled facilities) will be suitable if institutional placement is imminent. Both the Activities of Daily

Living Scale (ADL), developed by Katz, Ford, Moskowitz, Jackson, and Jaffee in 1963, and the Instrumental Activities of Daily Living Scale (IADL), developed by Lawton and Brody in 1971, measure clients' levels of functioning when performing certain tasks. ADL activities are: bowel and bladder control, ability to transfer, walking, wheeling, stair climbing, mobility level, toileting, dressing, bathing, and feeding. Clients are rated as independent or as needing assistance in each activity. Performance on the ADL scale indicates the type and amount of personal care a client needs. "Barthel's Index" (Barthel & Mahoney, 1965) is another scale measuring self-care abilities.

The IADL scale rates clients as either independent or as needing assistance with the following activities: taking medication, meal planning and cooking, housework and repairs, laundry, shopping, telephoning, money management, and travel. Monitoring changes in functional ability over time provides a significant indicator of the client's need for assistance. The client and family together can benefit from this evaluation, because it identifies needs that might have otherwise been overlooked. For the client and her family who are having difficulty in viewing their mutual situation clearly, those scales help to describe the client's abilities objectively. The "Hebrew Rehabilitation Center for the Aged Vulnerability Index" (Morris, Sherwood, & Mor, 1984) is a similar measure of daily functioning. Additional scales that blend MSQ, ADL, and IADL items are: "Functional Rating Scale for Symptoms of Dementia" (Texas Technical University, 1985), "Global Deterioration Scale" (Reisberg, Ferris, & Franssen, 1985), "Functional Assessment Staging of Alzheimer's Disease" (Reisberg et al, 1985), and "Clinical Dementia Rating Scale" (Hughes, Berg, Danziger, Coben, Martin, 1982). All these scales attempt to ascertain the effect of degrees of dementia on functional ability.

Support System: For most frail elderly clients the informal support system continues to be their major source of care and assistance. Long-term care programs should supplement this vital source of support; therefore, it is important for the case manager to understand the role of informal supports in each client's life. This domain describes the client's support or helping network: family, friends, neighbors, church, fraternal or professional affiliations, volunteers, and the nature and frequency of contact. This portion of the assessment also includes the recording of the client's living arrangements.

The case manager gathers information on existing formal or paid services received by the client, such as handyman, meals-on-wheels, or homemaking services. Case managers generally contact the main supporters, with the client's permission, to confirm information reported by the client and to discuss their perception of the client's status and how much assistance they render to the client. Spouses providing care are particularly vulnerable to stress related illnesses and may be frail themselves. The "Caregiver Strain Index" (Robinson, 1983) assesses the caregiver's feelings and stresses associated with caring for a frail, older adult. It has been well documented that social supports are often the key to an older adult's ability to remain in the community rather than enter a nursing home. The case manager must use support system information carefully when devising the care plan, knowing what care is or can be provided by informal caregivers and which supporters need respite from caregiving tasks. It is important to know who can go to the client's home in an emergency, and who is the primary informal caregiver for the client. The case manager's goal is to assist and strengthen the existing support system, not to supplant it with formal services.

Environment: The client's environment can present real challenges for the client who has functional deficits and wants to remain in the community. Actual hazards in the home, as well as the client's ability to maintain the environment, need to be evaluated carefully. The assessment includes a determination of the client's current living arrangements. The client's home should be evaluated for its current condition, hazards, and potential modifications. Issues to be considered include what access is there for handicapped individuals, such as, ramps, wide doorways, and railings on stairs. Also, how can the home be modified to accommodate the client's needs, modifications such as converting a ground floor room into a bedroom, equipping the bathroom with a grab bar or a tub bench, or modifying the stove so that the individual can reach the dials and stove-top easily. The client's subjective feelings about the environment are explored and may include such issues as: does the client feel safe there; can the client call the police or fire department, if necessary; can the client leave in an emergency; and, can the client easily leave to socialize with friends or participate in community activities. The client's environment may influence the care planning process. The client may live in housing where many needed services are provided and easily accessible, such as meals, housekeeping services, and a 24-hour emergency response system. Or, the client may live in a third-floor walk-up and have difficulty using stairs. Such a client may not be able to leave home to obtain care, and service providers may be reluctant to go to her home if the neighborhood is considered unsafe.

Financial: Financial information will help the case manager determine if the client meets eligibility requirements for publicly supported programs. In the financial area, the case manager gathers information on the client's income, assets, and expenses. This information assists the case manager in determining how well the client is managing available resources, her eligibility for other programs, and available resources should the client need to pay for some services. The case manager may need to spend time assisting the client with applications for public programs or helping to set up workable payment plans for past hospital and medical expenses that insurance did not cover. The case manager may even need to assist the client with construction of a budget. When the time comes to arrange the care plan, the case manager integrates information in this area with knowledge about available community funds, resources, and programs.

Table 3.1 contains an index to some commonly used assessment measures. No matter how detailed the assessment instrument, no single tool can provide all of the details of each client's unique situation. The case manager utilizes the instrument to identify specific issues and then, based on clinical judgement and experience, explores specific client issues to a

Table 3.1 Index of Measurement Scales

Domains	Goals	Population	Method	Authors
Emotional status				
Measurement of Functional Activities of Older Adults in the Community	Degrees of social dysfunctionality	Older Adults	Correlated social function with areas of need and cognitive/affective changes with social dysfunction	Pfeffer and Kurosaki (1982)
Cognitive abilities				
Brief Objective Measures for Determination of Mental Status in the Aged (MSQ)	Memory test to identify presence of chronic brain syndrome	Older Adults	Ten memory questions that indicate presence and degrees of chronic brain syndrome and associated psychosis	Kahn and Goldfarb (1960)
Short Portable MSQ	Mental status	Adults	Similar to MSQ	Pfeiffer (1975)
Folstein Mini-Mental State Status Exam	Mental status	Adults	Similar to MSQ	Folstein et al. (1975)
Cognitive Capacity Screen	Mental status	Adults	Similar to MSQ	Jacobs et al. (1977)
Set Test	Mental status	Adults	Testing ability to sort items by memory into four sets: fruits, animals, colors, towns—up to ten in each set	Isaac and Kennie (1973)

Zung Self-Rating Depression Scale	Mental status for depression	Adults	Assessment of affective disorder, especially depression	Zung (1965)
Functional ability				
Activities of Daily Living Scale	Evaluate functioning and assess need for care and response	Older Adults	Rating client's functional level: independent, intermediate, or dependent in personal care activities	Katz, et al. (1963b)
Instrumental Activities of Daily Living Scale	Evaluate functioning and assess need for care	Older Adults	Rating scale for functional levels: independent or dependent in instrumental activities	Lawton and Brody (1969)
Barthel's Index	Evaluate ability for self-care	Older Adults	Similar to IADL scale	Barthel and Mahoney (1965)
Hebrew Rehabilitation Center for Aged Vulnerability Index	Evaluate functioning	Older Adults	Similar to IADL scale	Hebrew Rehabilitation Center
Functional Rating Scale for Symptoms of Dementia	Symptoms of dementia and predictor of need for nursing home care	Older Adults	Combination of MSQ, ADL, and IADL type questions	Texas Technical University (1985)
Global Deterioration Scale	Severity of cognitive impairment	Older Adults	Staging system to assess level of impairment	Reisberg et al. (1985)

Table 3.1 ***(continued)***

Domains	Goals	Population	Method	Authors
Functional Assessment Staging of Alzheimer's Disease (FAST)	Evaluate functional abilities	Older Adults	Staging system specific to Alzheimer's Disease	Reisberg et al. (1985)
Clinical Dementia Rating Scale	Evaluate severity and range of dementia	Older Adults	Correlates with Short Portable MSQ to assess degree of dysfunction	Hughest, et al. (1982)
Social supports				
Caregiver Strain Index	Determine stress level of caregiver	Adults		Robinson (1983)

greater depth. This allows the case manager to develop a greater understanding of the client's values, what issues they want to deal with, and what interventions they are willing to accept.

Multiple Use of Assessment Instruments

The comprehensive assessment provides a method for identifying the client's strengths, weaknesses, and problems. With this foundation, the case manager can devise a care plan addressing the needs of the client within each of the previously described domains. The agency has relevant client data to utilize in evaluating existing programs and planning for the future. A comprehensive assessment assures continuity of care for the client and of case management services for the agency. It is important for the case management agency to develop guidelines for the assessment interview.

From a clinical perspective, the assessment helps the case manager understand the underlying cause of the client's problem(s) to determine if further evaluation or rehabilitation is indicated. When gathering data, the following considerations are important:

- Data gathered must be informative regarding the client's ability to perform routine tasks and her capability to complete entire tasks. For instance, a client might be capable of bathing herself, but be unable to step into the bathtub due to arthritis. If a case manager assesses a client in a temporary environment, evaluation of the client's usual living environment must occur.
- The data gathered should help the case manager systematically proceed through the problem-solving process with the client, by identifying problems and priorities expressed by the client and the informal supporters. The case manager shares assessment information with the client and informal supporters using language they can understand. Through negotiation, the care plan and goals are established. The case manager uses clinical judgement and experience to help the client in the decision-making process.
- Issues of clinical significance should be clearly identified and potential client risk assessed.

- The data gathered must be sensitive to changes in client status over time. In this way, the case manager can adjust services as client changes occur.
- The data should provide the case manager with an objective method of defining service category of need.

In designing objective measures of client status, the following conditions must be met:

- The client's functional status must be assessed using objective measures to minimize bias or manipulation.
- The questions must be asked in a manner consistent with the exact wording of the specific scales.
- The client's responses should not be influenced by the case manager.
- The case manager should focus on actual client performance, not on estimated capabilities.
- The client data should be verified through other sources, if necessary.

Case managers should be aware that while client answers provide valid self-perceptions, clients may tend to react defensively to some questions. Individuals may underreport physical symptoms or their ability to manage daily activities such as household chores, taking medications, or managing finances, because of fear of loss of independence. The client may respond, "Oh yes, I can cook all my meals," or, "I even prepare dinner for a friend sometimes," when in reality the client consumes only soup regularly. Or, the client may state, "Oh yes, I manage just fine on my Social Security check each month," when the electric bill is six months in arrears. She may also overreport family contacts and social outings, such as: "My daughter always takes me to church on Sunday and cooks me a meal afterwards," when the daughter actually visits one Sunday each month and brings doughnuts; or, "I just never miss the weekly bingo game at the Senior Center," when the client rarely visits the center. With the client's permission, the case manager should verify the client's responses. The case manager may contact other family members, friends, physicians, and provider agencies about their perceptions of the client's situation. Case managers may need to review past medical or hospital records, provider service records, and other correspondence. The more sources for information utilized, the more complete and useful the assessment data.

In some cases the initial assessment cannot be completed due to the client's condition. The client may be too ill to participate in the interview, or unable to communicate or be cognitively impaired. The case manager may use several alternative strategies. First, the case manager can obtain a "minimal client data set," asking selected questions, such as functional status, in order to develop an initial care plan. If the client is too ill to tolerate the complete assessment process, the case manager can divide the assessment into several sessions—collecting the clinical information in one visit, and returning to complete other sections on another visit. Another option is the "mini-assessment," in which the case manager assesses the client's presenting problems only. In this case, the case manager may consult with the client on critical problems which need immediate resolution through delivery of specific services. Another mini-assessment, the "branching assessment," allows the case manager to complete the mini-assessment, but adds particular trigger questions regarding more detail. For instance, if the client is being physically abused or neglected, associated areas may be probed by asking a series of questions:

"Why do you think the client is being abused?"
"Who do you think the abuser is? Why?"
"Are there physical signs shown by the client?"
"What is the client's affect? Afraid? Secretive? Defensive?"
"What is the family's reaction? Are they open? Secretive? Defensive?"
"What is the environment like? Does the client need help immediately?"
"Can the family continue to care for the client? Do they need respite? Counselling? Other help?" (Solan, 1986)

The case manager may ask the client to provide a "self-assessment." In this example, the client or the client's supporters will fill out the assessment questionnaire in advance of the actual interview with the case manager. This type of assessment may be useful when the client is very frail and dependent.

While all of these alternatives are possible and may provide adequate information for the case manager to begin the process of care planning, the author stresses that the optimal strategy is always to perform a comprehensive assessment face-to-face with the client whenever possible. All of the abbreviated assessment options increase the risk of an ineffective client care plan. The case manager is better equipped to develop an effective care plan when complete, comprehensive client assessment data is available.

The case manager must believe in the importance of the assessment process, as well as being skilled in the administration of the assessment tool. In certain situations, there is the danger that the case manager may hasten the interview process by eliminating sections if it is believed that the assessment instrument contains irrelevant questions. The case manager may decide to avoid areas that she or the client are uncomfortable talking about, such as sexual behavior or money matters, thereby missing important information. Or, the case manager may presume certain answers without bothering to ask the client the questions. Again, the case manager risks incorporating incorrect information into the assessment and threatens the integrity of the care plan. The case manager may withhold sensitive client data by not documenting the information. The case manager may justify this action as "protection" for the client. Case managers may employ other methods if they dislike the assessment instrument. Kane and Kane (1991) have coined the term "case manager's revenge" to describe these unorthodox tactics. If the tool seems too long and time consuming, the case manager might skip questions. If the questions seem awkward, the case manager may reword them. If the case manager believes the assessment hinders the development of a relationship with the client, the case manager may leave the tool in the car. If the case manager feels that family members answer for the client anyway, the case manager talks to everyone but the client. If the case manager believes that once they know the client well reassessment (regular review of the client's situation using a reassessment instrument) questions are redundant, the case manager may simply skip the reassessment process altogether. While very few case managers resort to such practices, it is decidedly in the client's and the agency's best interest to develop or utilize a user-friendly assessment instrument and to train case managers thoroughly on how to administer the instrument.

Nationally, several assessment instruments are available. All of these instruments are easily administered and use validated functional and cognitive measurement scales. Commonly used instruments allow for the transmission of understandable client clinical information between different health and community care providers, thus guaranteeing a continuity of information and care for the client. A listing and brief synopsis of some standard assessment instruments currently in circulation follows.

Sickness Impact Profile (SIP): This instrument is a multidimensional tool designed to measure sickness-related dysfunction in a population. This includes comprehensive, highly reliable rating scales, which can be numerically scored. The instrument can be administered in both oral and written formats. Although designed for the disabled population, the instrument can be used for the geriatric population. (Carter, Bobbitt, Bergner, & Gilson, 1976)

Older Americans Resources and Services Instrument (OARS): This multidimensional tool is designed to address three separate functions: clinical, research, and program analysis. This instrument measures functional activity in five domains: social resources, economic resources, mental health, physical health, and activities of daily living. The OARS provides information on functioning abilities and service need. (Duke University Center for the Study of Aging and Human Development, 1978)

Comprehensive Assessment and Referral Evaluation (CARE): Developed through a joint American/British project, this instrument was designed to provide information related to clinical syndromes and functional activity. Covering all domains and including a strong psychiatric component, CARE examines changes over time. The instrument uses a "branching" interview format, and flows smoothly during the assessment interview. (Gurland, Kuriansky, Sharp, Simon, Stiller, & Birkett, 1977)

Patient Appraisal and Care Evaluation (PACE): Developed by a consortium of four universities, PACE began as the Patient Classification Form. This instrument is multidimensional, objective, patient oriented, and relevant to patient outcomes. Critics feel that the psychosocial components are underrepresented and that it is not particularly helpful in guiding community placement decisions. (U.S. Department of Health, Education and Welfare, 1978)

Case Manager Skills

"The case management system stands or falls on the abilities of the case manager to perform the job" (Shueman, 1988).

The complex needs of long-term care clients are identified in the elements of the assessment instrument. Accordingly, the assessment skills of the case manager must be well developed. The case manager plays many roles for the client and for the case management agency: consultant, counselor, gatekeeper, data collector, problem solver, documenter, financial and service resource allocator, service coordinator, client advocate mediator, negotiator, service manager, and reimbursement overseer. (Grisham & White & Miller, 1983) A great many of these roles are inherent in the assessment process. While some skills are brought to the job through past education and experience, others must be learned through specialized training and continued education. A discussion of the skills the author believes necessary for effective case management is now presented.

First, the case manager must be *knowledgeable about the specific target population* served by the case management agency or program. In general, clients with chronic disabilities will include the elderly and other persons of any age afflicted with chronic functional or mental impairments. Case managers must understand both the aging process and human behavior. Professionals from the fields of social work, nursing, medicine, psychology, sociology, rehabilitation, public health, and other human service areas have the most training and experience. Involvement with persons with long-term disabilities requires a special sensitivity for dealing with the problems identified with these particular groups. Affected individuals struggle daily with loss of mobility, function, memory, friends, social contacts, and contact with the world—all of which deplete the client's sense of self-worth and productivity. One of the case manager's goals should be to encourage as much independence for the client as is feasible, in order to enhance self-esteem. To achieve this goal, the case manager may face an ethical dilemma: respecting the clients privacy and self-determination while fostering the client's protection and safety. For instance, older persons in urban areas may be especially vulnerable to crime. Can the client manage in this environment without risking injury to self? The case manager often walks an "ethical tightrope" with issues like the one described.

> *Alice was blind and everyone thought she belonged in a nursing home. She lived in the home she went to as a bride, and in which she cared for her husband until his death. She wanted to remain in these familiar surroundings. The case manager needed to assure her safety without increasing dependency in order to honor her wishes. The case manager contacted the state services for the blind who worked with Alice and the case manager to arrange for safety features in the home, which would assist Alice in preventing trauma such as burns and falls. A ramp to the front door was installed, so Alice did not have to climb stairs. Both Alice and the case manager were pleased with these solutions" (Connecticut Community Care, Inc., 1991).*

Second, case managers need to have *effective interpersonal skills.* Clients must be treated with respect and dignity. Addressing the client politely is very important. Even a simple amenity like using proper names, "Tell me, Mrs. Smith . . . ," reinforces the case manager's respect for the client as a unique individual. A partnership built on trust between the client, family, and case manager is fundamental to achieving positive client outcomes. Good listening skills are vital and will yield valuable information for the case manager. An older client may fear being "put away in a home" until she establishes a trusting relationship with the case manager. The client may prefer to reminisce about happier and healthier times instead of talking about her problems. The case manager must be prepared to listen and allow the client to verbalize her feelings and concerns, but redirect the client back to the interview at hand. If the client seems tired, the case manager should provide a respite until the client regains her strength.

Third, the case manager must have good *interviewing skills.* Case managers usually interview clients in person in their homes, but telephone interviews might be completed with family members, other supporters, and service providers. In each situation, the case manager must remain as a supportive listener, able to objectively deal with values and perspectives that may differ from her own. Skilled interviewers know that clients may tend to underreport certain conditions, and learn to ask additional questions to validate the client's statements. "You say you take four medications each day? Can you show me the bottles, please, so that I can write down the names?" The client may bring out eight bottles for the case manager to see. If the client's response does not seem to make sense, the case manager should also use observation to trigger additional questions. The client's environment can give much information regarding daily functioning. For instance, ask the client to give a tour of the home to observe any safety problems, barriers to mobility, or hygienic problems. Ask the client for a drink of water or accept an offered cup of tea to observe how easily the client performs simple everyday tasks. Through observation, the case manager can assess how the client walks and transfers, and even test the client's memory. Where is the sugar for the tea? Can she reach the cup and saucer? Is there adequate food in the refrigerator? Are the appliances in working order? Case managers must learn to communicate using special skills with sensory-impaired clients. For a visually-impaired client, the case manager may have to write information using large print, or write out questions for the hearing-impaired client.

> *Margaret lived alone in a small shack set back from the road in an isolated area. She was very cooperative in answering all the assessment questions. In response to the activities of daily living questions, she answered the case manager that bathing and personal care were not problems for her. As the case manager looked around the house, she saw an extremely cluttered home with little room for navigation. She could not see a bathroom in the house, but she thought that Margaret would object to giving her a tour. Instead, remembering that she had noticed a small shed out behind the house, the case manager asked Margaret, 'How often do you have to go to the outhouse at night'? Margaret replied, 'I use a chamber pot at night.' With this information, the client and case manager were able to discuss the disadvantage of not having a bathroom inside the house" (Connecticut Community Care, Inc., 1991).*

In this example, the case manager had used sensitivity and observation to help the client feel comfortable enough to talk about personal matters.

Fourth, case managers must be *knowledgeable about community programs and agencies* available to clients with long-term disabilities. Case managers should be familiar with eligibility criteria for existing community programs and the costs of services. Federal, state, and local programs can provide services and financing for eligible persons Such services include Social Security disability benefits, Medicare, Medicaid, Older Americans' Act Programs, Veterans' Services, Protective Services (for cases of abuse or neglect), housing programs, insurance, and many more. Case managers must be able to assist the client as indicated in applying to appropriate programs and to negotiate for the services to meet the client's needs.

> *Sally's son was incarcerated in a state prison 30 miles away. Her need to see her son on monthly visiting day was of primary concern to her. During the assessment interview, she continually reverted back to the loss of her son and her lack of transportation to visit him. The case manager was aware of a local church group who provided informal support to the elderly. She responded to Sally's concern by calling one of the members and arranging a monthly ride to the prison for Sally. After transportation arrangements were made, the assessment proceeded smoothly. Sally's emotional needs had to be addressed before her physical and functional problems could be assessed" (Connecticut Community Care, Inc., 1991).*

When dealing with family members or other informal caregivers, the case manager will often need to support them in their caregiver roles, and at the same time, not supplant their assistance. Case managers must be sensitive to signals from overburdened caregivers and provide services to provide respite for impaired caregivers, so that they may continue to assist the client in other ways. It is not unusual to have a 65-year-old daughter suffering from arthritis caring for her frail 85-year-old mother. The case manager needs to recognize the caregivers strengths and vulnerabilities.

Case manager experience can be beneficial when interacting with formal and informal providers of services. A case manager who has some history in dealing with provider agencies, especially within the medical community, often has an advantage over novice case managers. Good communication skills with physicians, hospitals, and home health agencies can ease a client into the health service network quickly. Physicians are extremely influential with clients and families, often directing them as to what type of long-term care services are needed and which providers would be most suitable to deliver the service. Case managers must be knowledgeable about medical terms and be ready to negotiate on the client's behalf with physicians for services the case manager believes necessary, especially if the physician holds another view. Physicians retain authorization over most medically related services (those that are reimbursable under Medicare, Medicaid, and private insurance). Home health care services, as well as most institutional services, require a physician's orders to deliver care.

Good telephone communication skills are essential in dealing with provider agencies as this is the most frequent form of contact. Provider agencies are contacted about mutual clients for referrals or information, such as arranging or changing services, monitoring service delivery, discussing a client's situation, and handling crisis situations. These contacts require the case manager to be sensitive to the provider's concerns while advocating for the client's needs.

Finally, the case manager must use good *time management skills*. There are constant challenges in admitting new clients, responding to clients in crisis, managing routine client follow-up, performing documentation activities, staff meetings, and supervisory/peer consultations, developing, professionally, and with other issues that take place within an organizational setting. The case manager is always reviewing priorities in responding to client's needs. It is especially important to be most efficient in clinical documentation skills and how to use the telephone to effectively assess the client situations.

It is important to note that the case manager must be committed to the assessment process. If the case manager does not believe that the assessment does what it proposes to do, she will not use it.

The case manager must believe that the assessment will produce the information necessary to complete the desired outcome(s) for the client (a suitable care plan to improve the client's living situation). Educating the case manager about the uses of the assessment instrument content, early in her employment, and proving its worth before it is used with a client, lends itself to commitment to the process.

In summary, the following client study illustrates an effective comprehensive assessment performed by an expert case manager.

Mrs. Smith had been admitted to a skilled nursing facility following hospitalization for a fractured hip. After a series of physical therapy treatments, she was returned to independence and wanted to return to her 100-year-old farmhouse. Mrs. Smith was 82 years old, a widow, with one terminally ill son who lived 1200 miles away. Her physician was reluctant to discharge her to her home. She spent her days pacing the halls of the nursing home, and wringing her hands in frustration. Mrs. Smith did have a younger neighbor who visited her at the nursing home, and this young woman decided to refer her to a case management agency for an assessment. Because the client did not have her own telephone, the case manager made an appointment through the social worker at the nursing home.

Present at the assessment in Mrs. Smith's room were the social worker, the director of nursing, the administrator of the nursing home, and the case manager. The case manager gathered information on her past and present illnesses and her current medications. Mrs. Smith was a diabetic and received daily insulin. Her vision tested 20/30, and her hearing was not impaired.

Emotionally, the client impressed the case manager as a strong individual who had coped well with life stresses. After her husband of 50 years became debilitated with Alzheimer's disease, she had cared for him at home as long as possible. When he was finally admitted into this same nursing home, she continued to visit and care for him every day. She either took a taxi or had a friend give her a ride, so that she could spend the day with him, feeding him and caring for his other needs until his death. The client now found it depressing to walk by his old room in the nursing home.

As they discussed her previous social activities, Mrs. Smith mentioned that she would like to resume attending Sunday church services. Several neighbors had helped take her to church in the past and also visited her at home before her husband's illness.

During the functional assessment, the review of activities of daily living verified that Mrs. Smith could ambulate with a quad cane, but was unable to climb stairs. She was able to transfer from bed to chair, but would need assistance with bathing. She had bowel and bladder control and could also dress and feed herself. Mrs. Smith was unsure if she could draw up her insulin, but she felt that she could inject herself. The case manager requested that the nursing home staff allow her to draw up her own insulin and inject herself on a trial basis. Her ability to do this would determine her need for skilled nursing care after discharge. The case manager also requested that Mrs. Smith be taught stair climbing, because the bathroom at her home was on the second floor. It was determined that Mrs. Smith needed help in all instrumental activities of daily living functions.

The case manager also evaluated Mrs. Smith's informal support system. Her only son was neither available or physically able to assist her at home. With her permission, however, the case manager called him to discuss Mrs. Smith's assessment, her desire to return home, and friends that she might be able to depend upon for assistance. The case manager contacted the young neighbor who had originally referred the client to the case management agency, and this woman agreed to do weekly shopping, manage her finances, be available for emergencies, and visit socially when she could. Two other neighbors agreed to continue visiting Mrs. Smith at home, and one also agreed to take her to church on Sunday. The case manager would contact the local home health agency to arrange for home health aid and homemaker service. Initially, the case manager set up meals-on-wheels to deliver lunch and dinner seven days a week, letting Mrs. Smith prepare a cold breakfast. The registered nurse would prefill the insulin syringes once per week if Mrs. Smith had difficulty performing this task.

The case manager had to assess Mrs. Smith's home environment. The client described her house as an "old farmhouse" with modern conveniences. The home was close to her neighbors. Although her bedroom was upstairs, she explained that she had taken to sleeping on the living room couch in recent years. Mrs. Smith felt that she could manage well in her home without making any structural changes. She was unwilling to install a bathroom on the first floor, but she felt that a commode would be acceptable. She did not really want to move her bed to the first floor, but agreed to do so if this sleeping arrangement was recommended for comfort and safety. The case manager and Mrs. Smith's neighbor arranged to meet at the client's home to determine what modifications were needed to make it safe and accessible for her arrival. Only a few changes were necessary: moving the bed and dresser down into the dining room, removing scatter rugs, and a general cleaning. Mrs. Smith agreed to all of these changes. The neighbor and her husband moved the furniture and cleaned the house. The case manager also contacted another neighbor's son, who agreed to do yard work, snow shoveling, and other odd chores for a reasonable fee.

Mrs. Smith's finances were assessed. She was already receiving Medicaid benefits, which would cover skilled nursing services once each week and home health aid, for one hour, twice each week for personal care. Neighbors and friends would provide shopping, transportation and socialization. The case management agency would pay for two hours of homemaking service once per week, and meals-on-wheels seven days per week. Mrs. Smith's Social Security check could be sent directly to her bank for deposit. Knowing that this banking process would take at least a month to initiate, the case manager asked her neighbor if she would be able to take care of Mrs. Smith's financial needs temporarily until the Social Security check cleared the account. The neighbor was amenable to this arrangement.

By the end of the assessment process, the nursing home staff agreed that Mrs. Smith could be transferred home after some intense therapy to teach her stair climbing and drawing up and administering insulin. After two weeks, when the arrangements were in place, Mrs. Smith went home for a trial period of three days. She felt comfortable enough after the trial period to remain at home. At this point, the nursing home officially discharged her to her home. The case mana-

ger had to adjust Mrs. Smith's care plan several times over the next two months, but she managed very well. Mrs. Smith remained in her own home for 18 months. After that time, she could no longer care for herself, and she returned to the nursing home, where she died six weeks later (Connecticut Community Care, Inc., 1991).

Care Planning

4

Care planning should reflect client goals and client needs. The best care plan in the world will not work if the client is not willing to follow through on it." (Connecticut Community Care, Inc., 1991) (After all, it is the client's care plan, not the case manager's or service provider's.)

There are three basic components of care planning. They are development, coordination and implementation, and monitoring and adjustment.

To develop a care plan, the case manager begins with the data gathered during the assessment process. The care plan is formulated in response to the assessment of the client's health, emotional, cognitive, functional, social support, environmental, and financial problems. Since the care plan reflects client goals and interests, the client and her caregivers must actively participate in its development. Through care planning, the case manager identifies all appropriate and available resources, including those in-kind services provided by informal supporters. The client care plan defines who will provide each service and the schedule, including the type, frequency, amount, cost, and payment source, of each formal service. A successful care plan is built on consensus between the client, caregivers (formal and informal), and the case manager. To coordinate and implement the care plan, the case manager first arranges for the prescribed services for the client by negotiating and contracting with both formal and informal providers of care. Family caregivers' responsibilities for care are determined and their tasks coordinated.

With the care plan in place, the case manager monitors the client's progress and makes any adjustments as necessary. Most importantly, the case manager makes sure that the client is satisfied with the service arrangements. As time goes on, the case manager continues to evaluate the client's situation for stability and any changes in the assessment domains described in the previous chapter. Based on this review, the case manager determines whether the care plan requires adjustments. In essence, the care planning process should:

- address the problems and strengths identified in the assessment;
- establish client-specific goals;
- develop a complete list of services to achieve these goals; and,
- explain the responsibilities of all the participants, the care manager, client, and informal caregivers and formal providers.

Financing mechanisms for care plan payment are varied and influence the case manager's decision about care types and amounts and will be discussed further. Also, case manager roles across the spectrum of caregiver and service reimbursement systems results in the case manager becoming a negotiator, family supporter, and client advocate. Finally, discussion of care plan evaluation and documentation requirements complete this care-planning chapter.

CARE PLANNING STEPS

The first goal of client care planning is to *develop* a workable *care plan,* and second, to *implement the care plan.* Care planning follows the assessment process, problem identification, and the exploration of problem resolution options, and results in the client, with information and guidance from the case manager, making the final decision about care options. Following the client's decisions, the case manager begins the implementation process by defining and coordinating the informal caregivers with the formal providers, negotiating the specific details of the care plan and arranging financing. When the care plan is implemented, the monitoring phase begins. The case manager provides ongoing oversight of the care plan, making adjustments as necessary in response to client changes.

Problem Identification

As explained in the previous chapter, the assessment process provides the case manager with comprehensive data on the client's health, functional status, cognitive status, emotional/behavioral status, support system, environment, and finances. The case manager analyzes this data and identifies problems and concerns. An active client problem list is constructed and the case manager develops possible solutions. The importance of accurate problem identification cannot be emphasized enough, because the best designed care plan is worthless if it is addressing the wrong problems. The following client study illustrates the importance of accurate *problem identification.*

Ms. A. is 62 years old, recently discharged from the hospital with speech difficulty and left-sided paralysis resulting from a stroke. She lives with her daughter and receives physical and occupational therapies, but she is not participating in therapy and is very depressed. The case manager interviews Ms. A. in her apartment.

Initially quiet and reluctant to speak, she grows more involved as time goes on. The case manager finds her to be very in touch with her own feelings of loss and anger because of the stroke and subsequent changes in her life. Ms. A. speaks of her depression and feelings of loneliness. The case manager helps her explore these feelings and emphasizes her remaining functional abilities. Together, they develop goals for care, which includes Ms. A working with her therapist to regain as much of her function as possible and receiving medical evaluation of a previously unidentified health problem. Ms. A. will begin mental health counseling to cope with her feelings of loss and changes in her life. Finally, Ms. A. will start going to an adult day care program to socialize with other older adults (Connecticut Community Care, Inc., 1991).

Problem Resolution

Solutions to client problems may come from a variety of resources. For example, the case manager may determine that the client's symptoms of depression are caused by the problem of social isolation. To solve the social isolation problem, the case manager has various options available that will increase socialization opportunities for the client. For instance, regular scheduled communication among family members, friends, and others in the extended support network could reduce client isolation. Or, the case manager might suggest community options like adult education, volunteer work, friendly visiting, or telephone reassurance to increase social contact for the client. Perhaps adult day care would be best, or maybe a companion service for the client, or a widow support group might be the best solution. Options vary and depend in great part on the creativity and experience of the case manager in identifying them and presenting them to the client.

Certain problems may stem from a client's special need. For example:

John S. is 78 years old and suffers from cerebral palsy. Cared for by his sister all of his life, he had never gone to school. He becomes very embarrassed when he cannot sign his name for the case manager. With John's consent, the case manager arranges for a literacy volunteer to meet with him regularly with the goal of having John be able to sign his name. When the case manager next visits John, he indicates that he wants to look at something in his record. He pulls out a form and proudly pens his name on the bottom. For the first time in his life, John had signed an official document without an 'X' (Connecticut Community Care, Inc., 1991).

An important aspect in seeking solutions to clients' problems is to involve all pertinent parties in the process. The more involved the client and the informal caregivers are in the process, the better the chance the case manager has in finding a logical, workable resolution.

Making Care Plan Decisions

Care plan decisions ultimately rest with the clients. To assist the client to make an informed decision, the case manager must discuss the pros and cons of all the possible options. Through this informed discussion, the case manager can guide the client as she selects the best alternative for her situation. When making care plan decisions, the client often relies on the case manager as the primary information resource. The case manager must be prepared to supply clinical information about health problems, available services, sources of reimbursement, and specific community providers. The case manager often uses negotiation skills with the client, the client's family, and other supporters to help reach a consensus on the most acceptable care plan. Care plan decisions are complex and clients may choose solutions that differ from a case manager's ideas of appropriate care. Although the case manager can try to persuade the client to move in another direction by offering more information, the case manager must defer to the client's right to autonomous decision making.

The client's final decision, however, should not be a measure of the case manager's success or failure in care planning. The case manager should be evaluated on the skills of assessment, developing interpersonal relationships, problem identification, knowledge of available resources, sensitivity to caregiver concerns, ability to communicate recommendations, and respect for the client's decision making. The client may choose not to follow the case manager's recommendations. If this happens, the case manager will have to be content with knowing that the process of case management was followed. The case manager then must decide whether or not to continue with the client and reassess the client's understanding of the recommendations, or wait until a future time when the client may be more receptive.

Care Plan Implementation

Once the client has agreed on a care plan strategy, the case manager begins the implementation phase. After the client has agreed to the plan, the case manager then begins actually arranging the care plan by exploring available services and sources of reimbursement. The two major tasks confronting the case manager at this point are coordinating and negotiating service providers and funding. Some areas may be rich in service resources, while other areas may be very poor in available services. The structure of the case management program may exert a strong influence on how the case manager arranges services and financing for the client's care plan. These two factors can be constraints to care plan implementation.

Clients fortunate enough to live in an area with many available services may have ample choices to meet their care needs. The case manager working in this rich service environment will spend time reviewing performance records and provider rates to select the most qualified providers. Sorting through multiple providers can become a challenge for case managers. It is tempting to revert to the same tried and true provider with the best record to save time and effort. Case managers must avoid complacency and retain objectivity when it comes to selecting service providers. Working within a team arrangement provides an advantage over working alone, because information can be shared with team members about new or less used providers who may be offering less expensive services with the same level of quality as established providers. Conversely, clients may live in a rural region, where providers are scarce and cannot provide a full range of services. The case manager working in this poor service environment will concentrate on leveraging all of the community and support resources possible in order to meet the client's care needs. This effort may result in improving the client's access to those few existing services, such as arranging transportation to dental clinics or to weekly physical therapy sessions. The case manager may also identify new, nontraditional resources and programs to fill the gaps in the service continuum.

Financing long-term care services can create a dilemma for clients and case managers. A deciding factor used to select providers may be the availability of funds to pay for them. The case management program's financial/reimbursement and service base influences the case manager's decisions when selecting providers and implementing the care plan. The case manager has greater leverage with providers who are paid or contracted directly by the case management agency than those providers who receive payment from other parties. The following examples describe how organizational models and financing mechanisms can affect care plan implementation:

Home Health Agency Providing Case Management. The case manager may have no authority to purchase home care services, but must rely on accessing insurance or entitlement funds like Medicare of Medicaid for client services. The case managers are most familiar with services their own agency provides and are aware of the financial incentive to use their own agency services first. Thus, clients may or may not be given multiple service options.

2176 Waiver Program, Nursing Home Preadmission Screening Program. The case manager has authority to use Medicaid monies to purchase community services not traditionally reimbursed by the Medicaid program. The clients have access to a broad range of health and support services directly through the case manager. The case manager acts as a gatekeeper for Medicaid funds. Usually, care plans are cost-capped at a certain percentage of comparable nursing home costs.

Social/Health Maintenance Organization. Pooled funds and consolidated services offer clients a full array of choices from acute to chronic care services. The case manager negotiates with health and social service providers in the organization.

The case manager is responsible for keeping care plan costs within fiscal guidelines.

Freestanding Case Management Agency. The case manager may have authority over a limited or large amount of funds for purchased services. The case manager depends largely on negotiation with providers to implement the care plan which may be financed through a mix of public and private resources. The case manager can be completely objective in arranging services, because her agency has no financial interest in the services being arranged. The perception of duplication of case management services can be an issue between direct service agencies and the free standing case management agency.

It seems the more authority the case manager has to authorize reimbursement, the less overall negotiating there is with service providers. However, increased funding authority requires that the case manager allocate those monies very judiciously. In some programs, the case manager becomes the gatekeeper for the funding source, by determining which clients, according to their disability level, are eligible to receive funds. For instance, in a preadmission screening program, the case manager must measure each applicant against a set of criteria for admission, while also making clinical judgements about the client's ability to manage independently. The case manager's assessment determines the client's program eligibility.

Gatekeeping does not always have negative connotations for the case manager. It can also be an efficient method for using limited resources in the most cost effective manner for the client and third party payor. The case manager bears a special burden of cost consciousness in those programs with a capped dollar amount for services. While some client situations may not be problematic, others will present difficult challenges. The case manager can be caught in an ethical dilemma where, from her professional viewpoint, budget constraints may no longer meet the client's care needs. In these situations, the case manager must be especially resourceful and try to locate additional funding or in-kind services to meet the client's care needs. In the Channeling Demonstration, case managers faced provider shortages when attempting to implement a care plan, so matching clients with scarce providers took on an added dimension. For instance, the case manager would assign a bed-bound client without any informal supports to a higher quality service provider than a similar client who lived with family members. The case manager reasoned that the family members in the latter case would monitor the provider closely, assist in the caregiving if necessary, and notify the case manager if problems arose. (Carcagno et al., 1986)

As a gatekeeper, the case manager can educate the client on how to use their resources to the best advantage and stretch dollars as far as possible without sacrificing quality of care. In the following example, the case manager, while advocating for the client, also served the best interest of the funding source.

A case management agency was involved with Ms. L. when she was temporarily placed in a nursing home, due to poor functional abilities and concerns for her safety at home. Medicaid would pay for the nursing home rehabilitation and stay, and even divert funds to pay her apartment rent, but only for three months. The physical therapist in the home did not immediately see her, waiting instead for written authorization from Medicaid for Ms. L.'s needed back and leg brace. The case manager, however, advised the nursing home to obtain verbal authorization from Medicaid in order to initiate Ms. L.'s therapy as soon as possible. Gaining such authorization, Ms. L. began therapy soon thereafter, and she was able to make good use of her time in rehabilitation. By acting to expedite procedures, the case manager served both the funding source and the client by saving the state expensive reimbursement for a lengthy nursing home stay and returning the client to her home in the community (Connecticut Community Care, Inc., 1991).

The next client example demonstrates how several services are phased in over time to the client.

Dolly T. was blinded by glaucoma 30 years ago. Since then she has depended on her family, her church, and Social Security for assistance. She has managed fairly well until recently when she found that shopping was too exhausting, because of discomfort from her arthritic hip. Hearing about a case management agency through friends, she called to request help with grocery shopping. After an assessment, the care manager identified several other medical problems needing further evaluation. First, the case manager encouraged Dolly to use a homemaker service to buy groceries and to do her shopping. Dolly had never worn dentures before, but a visit to a dental clinic convinced her how much easier it was to chew with them and improve her food choices. The case manager emphasized the importance of regular eye examinations, even though Dolly was blind, and Dolly returned for regular evaluation. The telephone was vital to Dolly, but it was becoming troublesome to use because her hearing had deteriorated. The case manager arranged for hearing tests that resulted in Dolly trying a hearing aid for the first time; thus, maintaining her connection with others (Connecticut Community Care, Inc., 1991).

CASE MANAGER ROLES ACROSS THE SPECTRUM OF CAREGIVERS AND SERVICE REIMBURSERS

The Case Manager as Negotiator

As stated previously, the care manager plays several roles with the client, the family, and the service providers during the care planning process. The primary role is one of negotiator between the client and the provider, and sometimes between the client family members. Another important role is one of client advocate. The case manager must be able to view the client as a participant in various life systems: the family system, the community system, and the health and human service system. From this perspective, the case manager's important role as a negotiator is easily recognized. The case manager negotiates on behalf of the client with government programs, formal service providers, and even the clients informal caregiving network.

Government Entitlement Programs

All of the government entitlement programs have their own eligibility requirements, application forms, and covered services. The following example illustrates some of the problems a frail older person can have with the health system.

Juan R. is 71 years old. A robust man, accustomed all his life to heavy work, he is now unable to climb stairs or carry large items. Emphysema has limited his ability to function independently in most activities. Living alone, with no family to assist him, he was referred to a case management agency for help with household tasks. The case manager arranged for housecleaning help and identified several health problems during the assessment process. Juan calls his case manager his 'mother and his lawyer,' because she helps him negotiate the health care system. After Juan had cataract surgery, he started to pay the surgeon's fee, because he never thought to mention that he had Medicaid coverage. The case manager explained to Juan what his Medicaid benefits covered and helped him to correct the situation with the surgeon's office. Later, Juan lost his glasses, called the doctor, but was told he had to wait three months for an appointment. When the case manager contacted the doctor's office, she discovered that they had misunderstood Juan: he was given an immediate appointment (Connecticut Community Care, Inc., 1987).

Formal Service Providers

There are a multitude of health and social service providers in the community. However, because of their service reimbursement mechanisms, they, too, like government entitlements, have eligibility and access requirements. Community services include:

- Skilled nursing service
- Home health aide
- Physical, speech, and occupational therapy
- Personal care attendants
- Homemakers
- Chore workers
- Companions
- Home delivered meals
- Emergency response systems
- Respite care
- Adult day care
- Psychological counseling
- Financial counseling

The case manager may arrange for a variety of services from several different providers in order to meet the client's needs. As noted earlier, selecting providers can be dependent on client choices, service availability, and financial resources. Some providers accept clients only if they are eligible for certain reimbursable program services. In the Channeling Demonstration, certain providers, even though they had previous contract arrangements with the project, still insisted on performing their own client evaluation to determine what services were necessary. In these cases, service prescription became a collaborative process between the case manager and the service provider. (Carcagno et al., 1986) With multiple providers, negotiation must be performed for each service provided. If funding requirements change, the case manager may have to discontinue a current provider's service and arrange a new provider; hence, introduce a new worker into the client's home. Although the client would have to consent to this new arrangement, the prospect of having to adjust to a new worker is not always easy. Throughout this process, the challenge for the case manager is leveraging funding for needed client services, linking clients with the most appropriate community services, and making sure that the client and provider are satisfied with the arrangement.

The following example demonstrates how a case manager must at times do more than simply arrange community services. In this case, the case manager used clinical expertise to persuade a reluctant housing authority to accept the client.

When Ms. L. was ready for discharge to the community seven months after her nursing home admission, the case manager helped her obtain an apartment for the handicapped in a new senior citizen's housing development. The case manager worked out a plan of care that included: family support with setting up the apartment and ongoing money management, friendly visiting, a homemaker, a home health aide, companion services, and ongoing case management. The housing complex was somewhat reluctant to accept Ms. L., because she was disabled and had not lived in the community for such a long time. The case manager had many contacts with the housing development's administrator, even writing a letter explaining the client's extensive plan of care, the client's mental alertness and determination to succeed in the community setting, the family's support, and the continued involvement of the case management agency. In the end, the thorough, painstaking efforts of the case manager paid off. Eight months after being institutionalized, Ms. L. was released to the senior housing facility (Connecticut Community Care, Inc., 1991).

Informal Caregiving Network

The informal caregiver network includes family members, friends, neighbors, church members, volunteers, and other community contacts, organizations, and clubs. This vital, caregiver network may include: the daughter-in-law, who performs countless services each day when she visits; the neighbor across the hall, who brings a paper over each morning; and, the distant relative who telephones once a week. A case manager considers the role of each of the informal caregivers first and negotiates with them on their ongoing role prior to using formal care providers. With the client's permission, the case manager discusses the client's situation with each supporter, verifying the assistance provided and assessing the caregiver stress. The case manager then ascertains whether or not some supporters do more than others and negotiates some delegation of care giving, if possible.

The areas of most frequently provided assistance by informal caregivers are:

- shopping/errands/transportation
- financial management/support
- meal preparation
- personal care
- housekeeping/laundry
- home maintenance
- medications
- arranging for benefits or services
- emotional reassurance/companionship (Scharlach, 1988; Sterthous, 1986)

Informal caregiving can require a significant commitment of time and energy. Studies have shown that women tend to help more with personal and household tasks, while men help more with home repairs, financial management, and transportation. Some caregivers spend an average of four to five hours per day, seven days per week, performing these tasks (Osterkamp, 1988). In the Channeling Demonstration, caregivers reported a higher rate of six hours per day in caregiving, but this project enrolled extremely frail, older adult clients (Christianson & Stephens, 1986). According to informal caregivers, the major problem that older adults face is isolation, especially as they lose the mobility and independence of their younger years, and they may experience loneliness and depression, perhaps for the first time (Sterthous, 1986).

The typical informal caregiver is a middle-aged woman, caring for her elderly relative in addition to having her own dependent children to raise, and who also may be employed outside the home. Approximately 75% of caregivers are women who are wives, daughters, and daughters-in-law. But, since less than 40% of women 65 years and older are married, the caregiving duty falls primarily to daughters and daughters-in-law. Of these younger women, 30% to 50% are also caring for dependent children. One-third of these caregiver women are 65 years old or older themselves. (Population Reference Bureau, Inc., 1990) Nearly one-third of informal caregivers are employed, and, of these, the majority work full time. Employers may have 20% to 28% of their employees involved in some kind of caregiving at any one time (Christianson & Stephens, 1986; Scharlach, 1988). With the increasing number of women entering the workforce, now over 50%, coupled with the fact that women provide the major share of caregiving, the informal support network faces serious a threat to its ability to continue this caregiving burden. Caregivers, once involved in this helping capacity, continue to juggle obligations even as their commitment to caregiving increases. As the older adult experiences increasing frailty and demands greater attention, caregivers tend to match the new requirements. Similarly, caregiving tasks will increase in intensity, becoming more difficult and unpredictable over time as the older adult's condition deteriorates. The wives of severely impaired men provide the most tasks and the broadest range of tasks involved with informal caregiving (Collopy, Dubler, & Zuckerman, 1990; Osterkamp, 1988).

The following example illustrates some of the burden of caregiving.

> *We have, for 5-1/2 years, been caring for our mother who is an 82-year-old stroke victim. She is completely paralyzed on her left side and is incontinent of bladder and bowel. The only function she can perform is feeding herself, which she does poorly. She requires complete care and is moved from bed to wheelchair by means of a Hoyer lift. My sister works and I have family obligations, and, as of late, have been plagued with some serious health problems of my own. Despite all these problems, and the everyday stress that goes into doing a job like this, we want to continue as long as possible (State of Connecticut, 1987).*

Caregiving for a chronically impaired person has its problems and its rewards. The act of caregiving is intrinsically related to personal health, morals, and philosophy, and is further complicated by its connection to the family. For the daughter caring for her debilitated mother, caregiving is not just a simple chore of cooking a meal, but a task performed out of love, guilt, obligation, kindness, sacrifice, or convenience. Caregiving is an open-ended commitment, which families may initially assume without understanding the full repercussions. Caregivers can overestimate their ability to provide care or underestimate the progressively disabling conditions experienced by the family member. (Collopy et al., 1990) Caregivers undergo intense emotional and even physical strain, to the point of becoming overburdened and unable to cope with the demands placed on them. Because of the time involved with caregiving tasks, caregivers give up time usually spent in other ways—with friends and family and at social events. For those caregivers assisting a cognitively-impaired adult, such as a person afflicted with Alzheimer's disease, the personal commitment is much greater than to someone without any cognitive impairments. These cognitively-impaired individuals require great vigilance, and their demands and at times unreasonable behavior can impose severe stress upon the caregiver.

Employed caregivers have a special set of problems. Due to the time commitments of both work and caregiving, these caregivers make significant personal sacrifices in their day. Some caregivers must decrease work hours or change work schedules in order to accommodate caregiving tasks. For instance, household chores may be performed before or after work hours or on weekends, but personal care tasks, such as bathing, dressing, transfers, and so forth, must be performed on the recipient's schedule. Losing work time and shuffling schedules adds pressure to an overstressed caregiver (Gonyea, 1987; Osterkamp, 1988). Caregivers may even have to take unpaid absences from work to fulfill caregiving responsibilities, such as transporting the relative to physician appointments and other places. Too many absences may result in a significant loss of income and may even mean loss of the job. Many caregivers experience poor health as they attempt to squeeze too many obligations into one day. Individuals would not participate in caregiving if they did not reap some benefits as well. To many persons, caregiving is a moral obligation. Individuals take on the caregiving responsibilities based on their love and devotion to maintaining the family. They may also assume that the family will repay this obligation by tending to their needs in old age. The following example illustrates the caregiving as a return of love and care.

> *Everything I am (or pretend to be) is a reflection of my beloved mother. My brothers and I were discussing her recently and our joint conclusion was that she was undoubtably the most unselfish person we have ever known. What was done for her was merely a continuation of what she had done for family and friends . . . she was the model for caring: bright and unusually understanding (State of Connecticut, 1987).*

Moral obligation to the community extends to helping friends, neighbors, and even strangers in times of need. Fulfilling such obligations can bring feelings of personal satisfaction and achievement to caregivers. Caregivers also report that by helping chronically impaired older adults, they feel that they are performing a very useful service and contributing in a meaningful way to the greater community. Finally, caregivers express satisfaction in knowing that the recipient is receiving adequate and quality care through their efforts.

Despite these benefits to caregiving, many families must finally turn to the formal system of services to assist them when the demands of the impaired older adult become too great. At this point, caregiver energy and finances are usually significantly depleted. Caregivers most often request help in the following areas.

Community Resources: What resources are out there that could be of help? Where are they located? How can we contact these resources?

Information about Aging: What diseases afflict the elderly? What are the conditions associated with aging? What are the psychological aspects to aging?

Patient Care at Home: How do you handle patients recently discharged from hospitals? Who can teach us how to perform more complicated health procedures at home?

Reimbursement System: How do we cope with all the forms and regulations? (Osterkamp, 1988).

By providing information and expertise in coordinating various services, the case manager can be supportive of the informal providers without usurping their authority or diminishing their caregiving responsibilities. The case manager's role with informal providers is first to assess their strengths and weaknesses through interviews and family discussion. If some caregivers are exhausted, the case manager can institute respite relief. The case manager's goal is to enhance the client's informal supports to allow them to continue to help the client. Informal caregivers are the most valuable resource the client has. In the Channeling Demonstration (1986), case managers were successful in maintaining informal service providers already in place. They had less success, however, in stimulating increased involvement among caregivers (who were presumably at their limits already), and in persuading other family members to join in a caregiving capacity. Case managers must be aware of problems that challenge caregivers and intervene to resolve those problems if possible. Resources for caregivers include counseling to decrease stress, respite services to allow freedom from caregiving obligations for a limited time, support groups to provide needed discussion and sharing with other caregivers, and medical referral to evaluate the caregiver's own illnesses.

When dealing with the informal caregiving network, case managers are often in the midst of intricate family dynamics. Many caregivers take their model for caring from another family member, embracing a parent's philosophy about caring, or are still wrestling with unresolved parent/child conflicts. Case managers must be sensitive to these issues when developing the care plan with the family. For instance, one family member usually carries the primary caregiving role for the impaired individual—whether because of proximity to the care recipient, or willingness to help, or a longstanding, close relationship with the person in need. This primary caregiver may feel resentment towards others who do not share the caregiving burden. Other family members may feel guilty about not participating in caregiving or believe that their relative is not receiving adequate care from the primary caregiver. Conflict over decisions about care are common. Family members may question the primary caregiver's decisions and wish to impose more of their authority on the decisions taking place (Collopy et al., 1990).

Because women outlive men, wives rather than husbands are more commonly the primary caregivers for impaired spouses. Spouse caregivers may experience a great deal of stress and suffer from their own physical impairments and stress-related disorders, such as ulcers and alcohol abuse. A spouse caregiver's health can deteriorate over time.

> *My husband had arteriosclerosis of the brain and is dependent upon someone to bathe, dress, and feed him. I have been doing this myself, but it is an awful strain. I wanted to keep my husband at home and care for him until such a time that I couldn't manage any longer . . . he couldn't be left alone at home. I couldn't get out of the house either (State of Connecticut, 1987).*

The parent/child relationship is played out during the caregiving situation. Parents have many irreplaceable losses as older, impaired adults: loss of friends, social groups, their homes, and their independence. Children retain a sense of obligation to parents to care for them as a debt for their upbringing. Yet, no matter how many tasks they perform, the children can never fully repay the parents. The ensuing anguish occurs when the parents express hostility towards the children (representative of anger over their losses), while the children feel guilty about their inability to keep the parents happy and/or restore their independence. In this scenario, the case manager must help the parents recognize and address their losses, through counseling or increasing socialization opportunities. The case manager must also help the children as caregivers see that they can only provide an environment good enough to maximize their parent's independence, and that they are not expected to manage, or be responsible for managing, all aspects of their parent's life (Berman, 1987). Care planning can clarify the obligations of the caregiver to the client and relieves some of the caregiver's guilty burden.

The Case Manager as Advocate

The case manager plays an important role as a client advocate. This is a natural role for the case manager, because of her relationship with the client and the depth of knowledge of the client's situation and preferences based on the comprehensive assessment. The case manager has much information to offer clients and their families, from client-specific care plan options, to a broad array of community and financial resources that are part of the long-term care system. This section will discuss ethical, legal, and care issues that may affect the client.

The case manager has the opportunity to discuss the client's right to make health care decisions and sign an advanced directive in the security of the client's home. The case manager should make the client aware of such options as living wills and advanced directives for health care. After discussion with family members and advisors, the client may decide to implement some or all of these documents. The client should be encouraged to share these documents with or express her wishes to her primary physician. The case manager must also determine if the client has or wishes to execute a last will and testament.

Another area where the case manager can be helpful to the client and family is in sharing information about the legal and financial issues associated with long-term care. These are complex issues and it is important for clients and their families to know as much as possible about these issues, such as Medicare's limited role in paying for long-term care services, and eligibility requirements for such programs as Medicaid. These issues may come up when the case manager is working with the client in developing the plan of care. It may be helpful for the client to know the actual costs of care and how the providers of this care are being reimbursed. The financial assessment provides an opportunity to discuss the client's options in funding her own long-term care services, should that be necessary. One of the common problems case managers encounter is having clients realize that the rainy day they have been saving for has finally arrived. The case manager can refer the client to a reliable financial estate planner, or help the client budget her own resources. Another issue of legal concern is conservatorship. Some clients may become incompetant and no longer able to make their own decisions or handle their own affairs. (Further information on conservatorship is discussed in Chapter 7, Specific Care Planning Issues.) If the client and the family discuss the possibility of incompetance, they can collaborate on a plan of action for the future. The client can make her wishes known about who should make decisions if she is unable to do so. Clients and their caregivers must also be informed about the client's rights to care, as outlined in the following:

- Right to nonharmful care
- Right to informed choice about care (costs, providers)
- Right to refuse care (may be part of care plan, but not necessarily all of plan)
- Right to fair assessment and grievance procedures (NCOA, 1988; Randall, 1989)

EVALUATION OF THE CARE PLAN

Once the care plan has been implemented, the case manager begins the monitoring and evaluation process. The initial care plan will likely undergo some adjustment over the first few weeks or months as the client and service providers adjust to each other. The case manager reviews the client's situation and care plan services to see whether the care plan is still meeting the client's needs. The case manager also checks to see whether the services are being provided as planned and if they are meeting the client's expectations. The case manager can evaluate the plan of care by telephone contact with the client, caregivers, and provider agency, by a home visit while the client is receiving the service (or a visit to the adult day care center while the client is there), by a review of written reports received from the provider, and as part of the regularly scheduled client monitoring contacts. Evaluation is a nearly constant process, closely integrated with the monitoring function. As the author discusses in the following chapter on monitoring, some clients require intensive evaluation because their condition is unstable, while stable clients are adequately followed by the regularly scheduled monitoring contacts.

DOCUMENTATION PROCEDURES

The comprehensive nature of case management services requires thorough documentation procedures. While documentation is usually not a case manager's favorite task, it is essential to establish accountability for the case manager's practice and to provide a standardized method of communication.

At a minimum, documentation should include assessment and reassessment instruments, the clinical notes containing summaries of these evaluations, documentation of all other contacts with or concerning the client, and a plan of care. The documentation should verify the client's eligibility for the program, the case manager's clinical judgements, and a clear justification of the plan of care. It is anticipated most agencies would provide for a client consent form and a bill of rights, and a fee agreement, if applicable. The documentation should be clearly organized, legible, and uniform. There should be established policies addressing the confidentiality and protection of client data. Client related data provide valuable information for program management, establishing personnel needs, caseload information, and formulating long-term policy decisions.

Clear documentation also encourages interchange of information between individuals and organizations involved in the client's care. Easily retrievable information about clients can be exchanged between professionals in different agencies. The case management agency benefits from using documentation methods that all employees understand. Staff in various positions may need access to information on the same client. Each staff member, whether another case manager, case assistant, supervisor, or auditor, should be able to select a client record and find what is needed. The following is a listing of possible forms to be included in a client record:

- Referral
- Bill of rights
- Consent
- Assessment
- Goals
- Assessment profile
- Clinical progress notes
- Service orders
- Fee agreement
- Reassessment instrument
- Discharge summary

Methods of Documentation

Most of the forms mentioned above are designed to fulfill specific information needs or service purposes. For instance, the fee agreement defines what payment arrangements have been made between the client receiving services and the case management agency. The referral form indicates how the client was referred to the agency. Three potential methods of recording progress notes are discussed below.

The first method is the narrative or "story" format. With this format, the client's progress is noted in a narrative style, similar to a story being related to another person. The case manager documents all activity and contact with the client. Entries are chronologically noted. This method is easily learned, but information may not be recorded in a uniform manner. Changes in care plans can be intermingled with notes on specific problems. It is difficult to retrospectively review this type of record or to systematically follow a specific problem chronologically without reading the entire narrative from start to finish.

Another method for documentation of client information is the check list or flow sheet. In this type of documentation, information is quickly entered into the record by event, such as, "Instituted home health aide service, twice weekly for one hour, to perform bed bath and transfer, Medicaid pays provider agency." The benefit of this type of documentation is speed. A problem with this format is the lack of detail concerning the reasons for initiating the service. The case manager fails to note any clinical judgements or justification for the service. In this example, case manager and agency accountability may be compromised.

A third method, and one which seems most appropriate to the client with long-term care needs, is problem-oriented documentation. With this method, the case manager writes a systematic account of the client's identified problems. Entries are chronological, but since they are cataloged by problem type, a specific problem can be followed over time. This method allows anyone reading the client record to focus on one or many problem areas as needed throughout the client history. One system is called the S-O-A-P format, with each letter representing a category of information. "S" stands for subjective information or what the client, family member, doctor, nurse, pharmacist, mailman, neighbor, or other tells the case manager about a particular problem. "O" means objective information, or the case manager's actual observations or examination results during the modified physical examination. "A" represents assessment, or what the case manager thinks about the situation and includes the case manager's clinical judgement and justification for the following plan. "P" is the case manager's plan of action, or how to alleviate, change, or address the problems through provision of service, referral, or further monitoring as indicated. All contacts with the client from the time of initial assessment are written in this S-O-A-P format. The client's plan of care should match the services noted in the progress notes.

CONCLUSION

After the care plan has been developed, arranged, coordinated, and implemented, the case manager begins the monitoring phase of case management. The initial stages of monitoring may involve several adjustments to the client's care plan as the case manager continues to refine her knowledge about the client and the support system. A well-developed care plan should be clearly justified and address documented client needs. A clear system of documentation provides a means to evaluate the quality of the case management process.

5 Specific Care Planning Issues

Case managers face many challenges in their daily practice. This chapter focuses on an array of specific care planning issues. These issues involve ethical questions concerning the care manager's responsibility, as well as the challenges presented by unstable health problems, informal support systems, and environmental and resource utilization issues. After each issue is discussed, a protocol for case management action is provided. These protocols were developed at Connecticut Community Care, Inc., Bristol, Connecticut, and are currently used by the case management staff.

ETHICAL ISSUES

Autonomy in health care decisions comes up again and again when discussing the frail, older adult. Collopy et al., (1991) state, ". . . in long-term care . . . [the] conditions of frailty and dependence on caregivers can severely threaten the self-determination of the elderly." Frail older adults may require additional support beyond family and friends, if they want to remain in their home environment. Receiving this assistance enables frail older adults to function as independently as possible and to enjoy a lifestyle of their own choosing (Clark, 1991). By acknowledging the existence of these opposing needs, autonomy and dependence, the case manager fundamentally empowers the client by organizing the community resources to meet the client's needs.

A pervasive ethical dilemma for case managers is balancing the older client's autonomy with state laws that require many situations to be reported because of the client's age. Case managers are trained to respect the client's autonomy in spite of deterioration of functional abilities and demands of family and supporters who may place safety concerns over the client's desire to remain in her own home. Yet, what if the client disagrees with the case manager's recommendations? What if the client refuses treatment that the case manager believes to be essential? What if the case manager feels the client is putting herself in a dangerous situation? Several major care planning issues and concerns, as well as state laws and public spending limits, may place the case manager in conflict with the client's autonomous decision-making. In situations of client incapability or serious self-neglect, state laws require mandatory reporting of specific situations and may abridge the right of frail clients to continued autonomous decision-making.

Conservatorship

Conservatorship is defined as the protection and care of the individual and the estate when the person is no longer competent to handle her own affairs. It is estimated that 80% of guardianship cases involve persons aged 60 years old or older. And, in 75% to 80% of these cases, a family member is appointed legal guardian (Bulcroft, Keilkopf, & Tripp, 1991). If a family member is not available to be conservator, other options may be a public agency or public agent, the probate court, an attorney, a case manager, or others.

Conservatorship involves a determination of whether the client can competently handle her own affairs. Case managers must consider the issue of capability if a client's refusal of services or professional advice places the client in imminent danger, and if the client does not seem to understand the consequences of her decision. The case manager must question whether the client is making a rational decision by examining the client's decision-making process, and the influence, if any, of the client's support system.

The case manager must evaluate the client's capacity for functional decision-making by determining if the client can rationally explain the reason for her decision, is aware of the alternatives, and understands the consequences of her decision. The case manager should also evaluate the client's cognitive status with a recognized test.

Other considerations are whether the client's decision will affect the well-being of another vulnerable person. In many cases, a client's decision may have a detrimental effect on a dependent spouse or other family member (Brostoff, 1988).

The client's support system can exert a powerful influence over the client's health care decisions. The case manager must evaluate the client's ability to make informed choices and determine whether these decisions are being disregarded by supporters. Under such influence, clients can become very passive, pliant persons, who do not believe that they have any options (Collopy, et al., 1990; Kapp, 1991).

After thoroughly evaluating the client's situation, the case manager makes a determination of client competency. If the case manager determines that the client is incapable, then recommendations should be made to the client's family or supporters about obtaining further evaluation of the client's symptom or about securing conservatorship. If client competency has been a long-standing problem and there is no one else to take action, the case manager may discuss her assessment with the probate court. The ultimate decision about competency is made by the legal system.

In some situations, there is no one to initiate the process or assume responsibility for having a client conserved. If the case management agency assumes this responsibility, there should be specific policies and procedures developed to guide the case management staff.

The following policies have been developed and are used by

the case management staff at Connecticut Community Care, Inc.

Before the organization initiates a petition for conservatorship, there must be the finding that:

- No other suitable person is available to act as conservator.
- The case manager must complete an assessment and attempt to have the client medically evaluated to verify the client's condition prior to acceptance of appointment as conservator.
- The case manager, supervisor, and director share in making the final decision to file for conservatorship.

Upon appointment as conservator, the case management staff observe the following protocols:

- The supervisor and case manager determine the appropriate schedule for client contacts.
- All staff members who assume "on-call" duties are made aware of all conserved clients.
- The case manager consults with the probate courts, and other appropriate individuals, when decisions are to be made regarding the client.
- The case manager seeks the advice of the probate court on any questionable situations, such as surgical procedures, "do not resuscitate" orders, or conflicts with the financial conservator.
- The case manager submits a report to the probate court whenever major changes in the client's situation occur, such as change in residence or surgery intervention.
- A copy of reports are filed in the client's record and regular reports are submitted to the probate court.

The agency's continued appointment as conservator should be reviewed on a regular basis. If this is no longer indicated under the following circumstances, a letter of resignation should be submitted to the probate court.

- The client improves and is found capable of managing her own affairs.
- The client moves out of the state.

- Another individual is identified who is able to assume the responsibilities of conservator.
- In other circumstances, with approval of the probate court.

NURSING HOME PLACEMENT

The decision that the client can no longer be cared for in the community and must be placed in a nursing home can be extremely difficult and emotionally painful. As noted earlier, no definitive method exists to predict who will need placement. Each situation is unique, with multiple variables to be considered, such as providing for the client's physical care needs and the client's cognitive capability. Studies have indicated that one of the most critical concerns influencing the decision is the availability of informal supporters, especially a spouse, to provide care. In one such study (Lieberman & Kramer, 1991), the highest incidence of placement occurred when the primary caregiver was a son or daughter. The stressed adult child who is the primary caregiver is most likely to choose placement when the client exhibits behavioral problems or there is a financial burden.

The case manager can provide emotional support and an objective assessment of the client's care needs, and find available resources to meet those needs. Many clients rely on their family and supporters to help them with the placement decision (Kapp, 1991). When the client's family, the primary supporters, and the case manager agree that nursing home placement is the most appropriate alternative, the client may still refuse. The case manager may then become involved in helping to resolve the dilemma. The case manager's first responsibility is to the client. The case manager must ascertain whether the client's decision is based on an accurate assessment of her ability to meet her physical care needs or is influenced by denial of her needs and fear of losing her home. By remaining at home, the client retains control over her own care and does not relinquish authority to an institution. A client's incapacity can also be camouflaged by her familiar home setting, established routines, and family support. An attempt should be made to determine if the client is making a rational decision even though her ability to manage at home is borderline. (Collopy et al., 1990) The case manager must offer her best professional assessment of the situation to the client and the family.

If the client has made a reasonable decision, and is aware of the risks of remaining at home, the case manager should accept the decision. In some instances, the client's decision means imposing a heavy burden on informal supporters who must respond to the client's care needs. These caregivers may genuinely want to honor the client's wishes, but be unable to meet the client's physical care needs, or lack the financial resources to purchase formal services. If at all possible, the case manager should attempt to support the client's wishes by developing a plan that utilizes all available resources (Kane, 1988; Kapp, 1991).

In assessing client risk, there are a number of situations that the case manager should consider in addressing care planning needs. Specific protocols for dealing with these issues are noted in Tables 5.1–5.11 at the end of this chapter.

Terminal Illness

Case managers may enroll clients when they are in the terminal phase of an illness. Besides the specific course of action dictated by the nature of the terminal illness, the case manager should discuss care options and where the client wishes to die with the client and family. The client should be made aware of her right to express her wishes in a living will, or advanced directive for health care.

Noncompliance or Refusal of Essential Services

There are clients who refuse treatment or care plan recommendations. For example, a client may elect not to take medications as prescribed or refuse personal care assistance. Although the client has the right to refuse treatment or care, the case manager should explore the refusal in a nonjudgemental manner to determine if there is additional information that needs to be presented about the consequences of the client's actions. Using a method similar to the one discussed in the conservator section, the case manager should assess the client's capability and capacity for functional decision-making. Some factors that may influence the client's decision include previously experienced side effects with the medications, or fear of strangers coming into her home. As Collopy et al. (1990) state, ". . . [the] client [is] unwilling to accept the increasing level of dependence in an environment where [she] once functioned independently." If the client understands the consequences of her refusal, the case manager must support the decision within established agency guidelines and state laws governing self-determination by older adults.

HEALTH PROBLEMS

Unstable Health Problems

Frail, impaired older adults may suffer from multiple chronic conditions that affect their daily lives. While some of these conditions can be stabilized, others may be so poorly controlled as to place the client's life in danger. If not dealt with on a timely basis, these unstable problems could lead to the client's deterioration or hospitalization. Case managers must arrange for these unstable clients to be carefully and closely monitored.

Increased Physical Care Needs

Clients can experience a sudden increased need for physical care beyond the limits of their original care plan. When the care plan is inadequate to meet these new, more demanding needs, the case manager must arrange to adjust the care plan to meet these new needs. This includes involving informal caregivers as well as formal service providers. These new adjustments may exceed the capacity of the informal supports or exceed public program cost limits and require a reevaluation of the client's ability to remain at home.

Emotional/Behavioral Problems

Clients may exhibit major emotional or behavioral symptoms, such as depression, or assaultive behaviors. These symptoms may be related to acute psychiatric problems or severe cognitive impairment that require immediate evaluation and treatment and also rapid response by the case manager to avoid placing the client or others in danger. It can sometimes be very difficult to secure adequate response to these serious problems.

Cognitively Impaired Client—Living Alone

The client who lives alone and presents evidence of cognitive impairment, such as short-term memory loss, confusion, or impaired judgement, can be a threat to herself and to others and must be carefully evaluated to determine the cause of the impairment. Alzheimer's disease, other dementias, post-stroke problems, infections, and metabolic disorders can result in cognitive dysfunction. Regardless of the origin, the case manager should carefully evaluate the degree of the client's cognitive impairment, request further evaluation from a physician or psychiatrist, if necessary, and document the impact of the problem on the client's ability to manage.

Substance Abuse

Substance abuse can be a well-hidden problem in the elderly population and should be considered when symptoms or behaviors cannot be otherwise explained. If the client acknowledges the problem and is willing to accept treatment, substance abuse problems should be managed as other physical problems. For example, if abuse is the result of taking medication improperly or of addiction to pain killers or alcohol, the case manager can take appropriate action to assist the client. Continued substance abuse can put the client at risk of developing more serious health problems.

INFORMAL SUPPORT SYSTEM ISSUES

Unstable Informal Support System

At times, the client's informal support system can break down, leaving the client without necessary care. Supporters can suffer from overly burdensome demands and find that they are unable to continue in their caregiving roles. They may be unwilling to perform caregiving functions any longer and have no one available to replace them. Clients also may not have an adequate number of informal supporters to assist them with their care. All of these situations may result in the failure of the informal support system. The client's needs can change dramatically, placing an increased burden on a support system that cannot handle the new demands. The support system itself may change. Primary caregivers may become ill, leave the area, or experience the consequences of extreme stress, such as exhaustion, depression, or a deteriorating relationship between the client and the caregiver. The case manager must evaluate the extent of the support system failure, and offer immediate help, if possible, to relieve the stress. In these situations, the case manager must be sensitive to the role of family dynamics (Selig, Tomlinson, & Hickey, 1991). The case manager may suggest respite services to decrease the caregiving burden or counseling sessions for caregivers to relieve their emotional stress. If alternative care resources are not available, the case manager may have to recommend temporary or permanent institutional placement for the client.

Abuse

Abuse is defined as neglect, exploitation, and verbal or physical insult to the client. Neglect can take the form of intentional avoidance of caregiving duties that results in the deterioration of the client's health, or neglect stemming from ignorance, where the caregiver believes that she is taking adequate care of the client, but does not know how to provide proper care. In both cases, the neglect jeopardizes the client's health. The case manager must determine the nature of the neglect and proceed to act in the client's best interest.

The case manager must be careful to preserve the client's autonomy when exploring alternatives for care in situations of abuse. In some instances, the client may refuse to acknowledge family abuse or refuse to take steps to stop it from happening. Whatever options the case manager considers, the primary concern must be the client's safety. The case manager may be caught in a dilemma if the client is overly influenced or coerced by the family into believing that their care is not abusive in nature. When caregivers are being abusive from the case manager's viewpoint, but the family feels that they are doing the best they can under the circumstances, the case manager needs to work with the family in a sensitive and nonjudgmental manner. The case manager may be limited if the client refuses to acknowledge the abuse and the family is unwilling to change. The case manager must attempt to balance the client's rights (e.g., right to nonharmful care), while attempting to protect her from abuse.

ENVIRONMENTAL ISSUES

Uninhabitable Home

Some clients may be living in residences that are in such poor condition that they are virtually uninhabitable. The building may be in violation of housing or sanitation codes, or present hazards to others sharing the same structure (e.g., an apartment building or complex). If the client is unwilling to relocate, then possibilities for correction must be explored to respond to the housing problem. Some issues to consider include: is the client willing to act to correct the problems or to allow others to correct them; or, is the problem impossible to correct because the structure is too deteriorated physically; or, are financial resources unavailable to improve the situation. The case manager again must put the client's safety first and explore all community options in an attempt to ameliorate the housing situation.

In conclusion, as the number of very frail clients increases, the greater the likelihood of the case manager encountering one or more of these difficult and challenging issues. The case manager should always consult with a supervisor on these issues, as they may present risk management challenges as well as quality of care challenges to the agency. In order to create a framework for action, protocols like the ones that follow in Tables 5.1–5.11 can be developed to assist case managers in responding to the clients with these special needs.

Table 5.1 Ethical Issues: Refusing Placement

Definition	Client Characteristic	Case Manager Actions
Client has care needs that cannot be met by the informal support network and formal services.	Program resources are no longer adequate to meet the client's care needs.	Bring to the attention of supervisor. Evaluate client's cognitive status and continued capability—if client appears no longer capable, encourage informal supporter to begin conservatorship or if no informal supporter, initiate on client's behalf. Arrange conference with client/primary informal supporter to explore client's care needs and available options. If client continues to refuse placement, offer counseling to guide client through ongoing review of decision and alternatives. If client remains capable and is at risk, follow referral to Ombudsman/Protective Services guidelines.

Table 5.2 Unstable Health Problems

Definition	Client Characteristic	Case Manager Actions
Client is symptomatic and the symptoms are uncontrolled or not well controlled.	Client's symptoms are likely to lead to further deterioration and may require hospitalization. Examples of uncontrolled or poorly controlled symptoms are: sudden onset of confusion or unusual behavior; deterioration of functional status; increased difficulty in breathing; increased lower extremity edema; increase in pain; sudden onset of incontinence; or increase in frequency of falls.	Bring to attention of supervisor. If client followed by social service case manager, there will be consultation with a nurse case manager. Arrange for further evaluation in most appropriate manner, i.e., emergency room. Refer to primary medical provider or recommend evaluation by specialist. If indicated, contact informal support and/or emergency contact, concerning medical evaluation, arrange for ongoing follow-up by registered nurse from home health agency with monitoring parameters clearly defined.

Table 5.3 Increased Physical Care Needs

Definition	Client Characteristic	Case Manager Actions
Client has experienced *increased need* for physical care requiring significant adjustment of the plan of care.	Client has deteriorated and is *now experiencing* one or more of the following: existing skin lesion or high risk of developing secondary to immobility; inability to walk or transfer without the assistance of another person; inability to change position in bed or chair; inability to cleanse self after episode of incontinence; inability to feed self; repeated falls.	Bring to attention of supervisor. If client followed by social service case manager, there will be consultation with a nurse case manager. Arrange for evaluation of cause of increased physical care needs an potential rehabilitation. Determine if informal supporters have needed skill level to provide for client's care. Evaluate increased assistance by informal supporters and formal providers to meet client's increased needs. Communicate everyone's role in plan of care to all involved.

Arrange for registered nurse from home health agency to evaluate increased plan of care. If increased services cannot meet client's needs, explore alternate care options with client/informal supporters.

Table 5.4 Cognitive Impairment-Living Alone

Definition	Client Characteristic	Case Manager Actions
Client is cognitively impaired and lives alone.	Client lives alone and is presenting any one or combination of symptoms—short term memory loss, confusion, impaired judgement, or behavioral problems.	Bring to attention of supervisor. Carefully evaluate the degree of impairment and impact on client's ability to manage—personal care (especially bathing and dressing), household management(cleaning, laundry, meal preparation, and shopping), transportation, financial management, evidence of wandering or inappropriate behavior (check with family, neighbors, friends as indicated), ability to summon assistance in case of emergency. Conference with client/primary informal supporter to establish care plan, criteria for institutionalization, short/long term goals.

Short-term—determine if indicated medical evaluation has been obtained, help client maintain current cognitive abilities as much as possible, monitor for further decline.

Long-term—establish plan for when client can no longer live alone.

Table 5.5 Emotional/Psychiatric Problem

Definition	Client Characteristic	Case Manager Actions
Client is exhibiting major emotional or behavioral symptoms in the absence of any symptoms of confusion.	Client is demonstrating one or more of the following symptoms or behaviors: depression, talk of suicide, anxiety, hallucinations, assaultiveness, inappropriate sexual references, or other behaviors threatening to self or others.	Bring to attention of supervisor. If client is followed by nurse case manager, there will be consultation with a social service case manager. Determine history of emotional problems and past treatment by counselor or psychiatrist. Evaluate current symptoms/ behaviors. Suicide threat should receive immediate attention for evaluation by crisis team, counselor or psychiatrist, involuntary commitment may be indicated. For non life threatening situations, determine client's receptiveness to counseling or psychiatric evaluation.

Table 5.6 Informal Support System-Unstable Informal Support System

Definition	Client Characteristic	Case Manager Actions
Client's needs have changed to render her/him dependent on an informal support system that is no longer adequate. OR Client's informal support system has changed secondary to illness, emotional stress (i.e., caregiver exhaustion), or increased demands from others. OR The informal support system members remain or have become severely stressed by their care taking responsibilities.	The informal support system is evidencing severe stress and is at risk of breakdown and can no longer provide the assistance needed in conjunction with formal services to meet the client's care needs.	Bring to attention of supervisor. Evaluate for possible alternatives to relieve or restore the informal support system. Review program resources to increase assistance from formal services. Explore client's use of financial resources to supplement existing informal/formal assistance. Provide information on family counseling resources. Assess risk of abuse toward client/other family members.

Table 5.6 ***(continued)***

Definition	Client Characteristic	Case Manager Actions
		Arrange a meeting with client and informal supporters to discuss supporter's stress and client care options, including client's ability to remain at home.
		If issue can only be resolved by client placement, begin work with client on dealing with this issue.

Table 5.7 Refusing Essential Services

Definition	Client Characteristic	Case Manager Actions
Client is in need of essential services (physical care, nutrition, environment) to remain safely in home.	Client is refusing the case manager's recommendation of essential services.	Bring to the attention of supervisor.
		Evaluate client's reasons for refusing services.
		Evaluate client's capability and emotional status.
		Enlist aid of informal supporters to encourage client to accept essential services.
		Offer counseling if indicated to work with client on reasons for refusal.
		Evaluate safety issues.

Table 5.8 Terminal Illness

Definition	Client Characteristic	Case Manager Actions
Client is in the terminal phase of his or her illness.	Client is expected to die within 60 days.	Bring to attention of supervisor. If client is followed by social service case manager, there will be consultation with a nurse case manager for physical care needs. Project care needs over the next 60 days, assuming increasing weakness and disability. Identify specific care needs in reference to skin care, nutrition/hydration, elimination, pain control, emotional response, spiritual needs and informal support system. Determine if client is receptive to hospice referral. Make client/family aware of community/institutional hospice resources.

Table 5.9 Substance Abuse

Definition	Client Characteristic	Case Manager Actions
Client's substance abuse is having adverse behavioral or physical consequences.	Client may be known or suspected of substance abuse or is known to be actively abusing the susbtance.	Bring to attention of supervisor. If client is followed by nurse case manager, there will be consultation with a social services case manager. Identify issue to client in a nonjudgmental manner with observation of how substance abuse is affecting behavior or physical functioning. Advise client of substance abuse counseling resources available and assist as indicated. Advise indicated informal supporters of substance abuse counseling resources available, i.e., Alcoholics Anonymous.

Table 5.9 ***(continued)***

Definition	Client Characteristic	Case Manager Actions
		Arrange for monitoring of prescription medications if they are being abused.
		Advise formal providers, i.e., home health aide, homemaker, or companion, that alcohol products are not to be purchased for client.

Table 5.10 Environmental Issues: Uninhabitable Home

Definition	Client Characteristic	Case Manager Actions
Client's home of choice (moving is not an option client chooses) is in such poor condition as to be uninhabitable, be in violation of applicable housing/sanitation codes, or create a hazard or pose significant risk to others sharing same structure, i.e., apartment building.	Client does not appear to be willing to allow correction of the enviornmental problem, or the situation is too severely deteriorated to correct or would require financial resources that are not available.	Bring to attention of supervisor. Explore reasons for client's refusal of services. Evaluate client's cognitive status to determine capability. Determine if counseling is indicated to assist client with decision making process. If housing is rented, determine if assistance of landlord can be obtained to persuade client to accept correction of hazard. If housing is owned, determine if assistance of local housing inspector or health department can be obtained to persuade client to accept correction of hazard. Explore all possible financial resources to correct problem.

Table 5.11 Question of Abuse

Definition	Client Characteristic	Case Manager Actions
Client is being subjected to neglect, abuse, or exploitation.	Client demonstrates evidence of emotional or physical abuse, appears to be neglected by responsible caregiver or to be subjected to exploitation, or appears at high risk or any of these events.	
	Client may deny that abuse is taking place.	
	Bring to attention of supervisor.	
	Evaluate client for evidence of abuse:	
	Physical—bruising, pattern of frequent injury;	
	Emotional—appears fearful, passive, eluctant to discuss relationship with suspected abuser;	

Exploitation—there is significant change in financial resources without plausible explanation;

Suspected abuser describes extreme stress or denies stress in an obviously stressful situation.

Follow protocols in alerting the Ombudsman and follow-up with Protective Services.

Alert formal providers to monitor client for evience of physical abuse as indicated.

Offer counseling to client to deal with situation.

Offer counseling resources to suspected abuser.

6 Monitoring and Evaluation

After assessing the client and arranging the care plan, the case manager continues to evaluate the client's condition and the quality of the provided services. The care plan may require some revision, such as adjusting service hours, reviewing the responsibilities of informal supporters, or using discretionary funds to pay for a service temporarily until an entitlement program provides payment. Appropriate monitoring of the care plan requires regular contact with the client, family, and service providers. The case manager draws on her education and experience to determine the frequency and type of contact. Clients and informal supporters must feel comfortable about contacting the case manager with concerns or problems related to the care plan.

Each case management program should develop formal policies concerning the frequency of monitoring contacts. In general, programs establish standard time periods for client care plan reviews and the reassessment. At these prescribed intervals, case managers or other case manager support staff will contact the client, family, primary supporters, or formal providers. The purpose of these contacts is to evaluate the client's status, and the adequacy of the current plan of care, and adjust the plan of care as indicated by any changes in the client's condition or in the availability of the informal supporters. Unscheduled contacts between the client/family and formal provider may occur as the client's needs change. The degree of client frailty and the complexity of care may influence how much time and effort the case manager must invest in monitoring. Very frail clients require frequent monitoring, because their needs can change rapidly, and, if not attended to promptly, may suddenly develop into a crisis. The monitoring phase of case management will be discussed in two parts: monitoring methods, including formal and unscheduled contacts, and reassessment and evaluation of the care plan; and, provider relations, including the evaluation of the quality of delivered services. Within this framework, case managers, supervisors, and administrative staff work together to evaluate the client's plan of care and the service provider's performance. Thus, the monitoring process extends beyond the internal policies of the case management agency to an objective evaluation of the formal external service delivery system.

MONITORING METHODS

Formal Reviews

After assessment, the client's situation is formally reviewed at established, regular intervals. These scheduled reviews involve contact with the client, the family, and the service provider(s), and range from monthly telephone contacts to annual home visits. These contacts are made by case managers or case manager support personnel trained in the use of the review protocol. During these formal reviews, the case manager determines if there is any change in the client's condition and if the change requires an adjustment of the care plan. The case manager reviews the client's plan of care, making certain that prescribed services are being provided, and determining that the client and family are satisfied with the service. If the case manager finds there are changes in the client's status, these changes are discussed with the client, family, and service providers. It is important to review any identified problems with the client and all involved with her care.

For instance, if the most immediate problem seems to be under control, the case manager might suggest dealing with other problems that were identified during the assessment process. Again, these formal reviews are intended to make certain the care plan continues to meet the client's needs. The case manager also reinforces the importance of the client, family, or providers to contact her with any client problems or changes immediately, rather than to wait for the next formal review.

Reassessment

The reassessment is a formal review that is conducted at regularly scheduled intervals, usually six months to one year after the initial assessment. The reassessment is an in-depth, systematic review of the client's situation designed to detect any changes and to provide a complete updating of the client in all of the assessment domains. The reassessment instrument is modeled after the assessment instrument in order to allow for an accurate comparison and reevaluation of the clients status. Like the assessment interview, the case manager conducts the reassessment interview during a face-to-face visit with the client in the home or community setting. During the reassessment process, the case manager speaks with all of the client's formal and informal providers to review the client's situation and to learn about any changes that the providers may have noticed. The case manager schedules an appointment with the client and requests that any needed information, such as financial data, be available at the visits. The case manager arranges for significant family members or other persons to be present during the interview, as necessary. An overview of the areas covered in the reassessment process follows.

Meeting the client again requires time to get reacquainted and reestablish rapport. The case manager should review the purpose of the visit. The face-to-face visit provides an opportunity to objectively evaluate the client and her environment.

The case manager reviews the seven domains originally covered during the initial assessment. This data may be given by the client or the family or other supporters caring for the client. The reassessment domains are:

Health: Note is taken of new illnesses or incidents and resolution of previous problems using the initial health profile as a measurement guide. A detailed review of all of the client's current medications, including the dosage and frequency, is recorded.

Functional Status: Activities of daily living and instrumental activities of daily living are reviewed, and any changes noted.

Cognition: A review of cognitive abilities and any changes are documented.

Behavior/Emotion: Client's feelings and behaviors are evaluated.

Support System: Any changes, problems, or requests of caregivers are noted.

Environment: A review of living arrangements is made and the condition of the client's environment is noted.

Finances: Any changes reported by the client or her supporters in income or expenses are recorded. Fee arrangements and entitlement eligibility benefits are reviewed.

The case manager reviews the client's satisfaction with the plan of care. The case manager also reviews life events with the client since the last assessment visit, discussing any life changes or crises that have occurred. The case manager documents all client information gathered, comparing it with prior information and her objective observations. The nurse case manager will perform another modified physical examination, based on her observation or client complaint. The case manager analyzes all of the available data and shares her impressions and concerns with the client and supporters. They discuss client strengths, positive gains, ongoing problems, and any recent changes. Finally, the case manager, the client, supporters, and appropriate others decide on what interventions or care plan changes, if any, are necessary. Available options are discussed. The case manager then completes the interview by summarizing the actions to be taken as a result of the reassessment, the ongoing plan of care, and her next planned contact.

After the reassessment visit, any changes in the care plan are arranged by the case manager by contacting the service providers and negotiating the changes. The case manager also plans a follow-up contact to evaluate the new care plan. The reassessment instrument becomes a permanent part of the client's record. The case manager will then have a basis of comparison when the next reassessment is due.

Informal or Unscheduled Contacts

Unscheduled contacts and face-to-face visits are based on significant changes in the client, support system, or formal providers, and can occur at any time. These contacts are characterized by frequent interaction with the client or family or providers to evaluate the client's status and the triggering problem. The initial contact may come from anyone involved with or concerned about the client's care. Communication may occur via the telephone, a personal visit, a letter or report, or a multidisciplinary client conference.

Unscheduled contacts and visits usually occur because of a significant change in the client's condition. This change usually requires an alteration in the client's care plan. For instance, if a client requires hospitalization, the case manager should be involved immediately. Any institutionalization means termination of all current community services, and continuing contact with the client, the family, and the institution until the client is ready for discharge. Prior to discharge, the case manager must reassess the client using information from the staff, the family, and the client, and then arrange a new care plan.

Some client's conditions are constantly changing, requiring intensive monitoring, while other clients conditions are stable and are maintained with routine monitoring. The Channeling Demonstration (Carcagno et al., 1986) experience demonstrated that a proportion of the caseload experienced frequent crises. Crises may be family or client related, such as a primary caregiver being ill, leaving the client temporarily without regular care; or, a client suffers with unstable health conditions and needs continual service changes. Changes may be related to provider problems with staff shortages, turnovers, or reimbursement, leaving clients without adequate care. Case managers may spend a disproportionate amount of time on clients in crisis. Conversely, client situations can be stabilized as demonstrated by the following client example.

When she was 18 years old, Jody was involved in a motor vehicle accident. She suffered traumatic brain injury. After 12 years of hospitalization and intensive rehabilitation, she was ready to live independently again. Referred to a case management agency, she needed an unusual mix of services: first, some structured assistance to relocate, and later, much ongoing, flexible oversight to assist her adaptation to her new surroundings. The case manager helped her find an apartment and then located appropriate persons to retrain Jody in the necessary, practical skills of independent living: how to ride a city bus, how to go shopping, how to manage her finances, and how to plan her daily routines. The case manager arranged home care services to teach Jody when and how to contact physicians or hospitals for health needs, and arranged for a vocational trainer to assist her in finding employment. After this initial adjustment period, Jody's situation became quite stable. She contacted the case manager if she was frustrated by events or needed help. After approximately two years of ongoing case management, Jody was living independently with minimal home care services and case management services were discontinued (Connecticut Community Care, Inc., 1987).

Caseload Size and Composition

Client caseload size and composition are critical factors influencing the case manager's ability to effectively respond to client's changing needs. The type of client each case manager is responsible for varies from those that require routine monitoring to those requiring frequent and intensive interventions. A number of factors influence the number of clients a case manager can manage. For instance, a case manager in a broker-model organization may be able to manage a larger number of clients than a case manager in a comprehensive case management agency, because there are minimal monitoring tasks in the former model. The case manager's authority to purchase services can affect the client-caseload size. Case managers with authority to pay for services have an easier time arranging services, and less time is spent negotiating for the reimbursement of service providers. Another factor is the size of the geographic area covered by the case manager. A rural region may require extensive travel to visit clients, and take time away from other case management tasks. Dealing with very frail clients will require significant case manager time.

When first referred to the case management agency, Ms. L. was dependent in most activities of daily living and all instrumental activities of daily living. She had trouble with urinary continence. She transferred and walked with difficulty. She lived in a walk-up apartment, but could not climb the stairs without help. Her sister was living with her temporarily to assist her, but the two women argued continually. The case manager sought nursing home placement immediately to provide a safe environment to support her many functional deficits. After an eight month nursing home stay, Ms. L. was ready to try and return to the community. The case manager helped Ms. L. find a handicapped equipped apartment in a senior citizen housing complex, and arranged an extensive plan of care involving family support, home health aide, companion services, and ongoing case management. Case management services continued for four years. There were many incidents requiring case manager intervention. Three particular episodes are illustrated:

Ms. L. wore a heavy back brace to help her walk. Her new apartment faced south and was usually very warm during the summer, and the heat made her brace extremely hot and un-

comfortable. The case manager located a charitable foundation that was willing to donate an air conditioner for Ms. L.'s apartment.

Ms. L. found it difficult to live on her own. On two occasions, she panicked and could not function by herself. The case manager helped arrange a temporary nursing home stay after each incident. When the client indicated her interest in returning to her apartment, the case manager discussed both the pros and cons of living in an institution versus living in the community. They talked about the consequences of her emotional status and her panic behavior and its impact on her functional ability. Ms. L. chose to return to her apartment.

On another occasion, the volunteer who delivered Ms. L.'s meals-on-wheels called the case manager with the disturbing information that Ms. L. was talking about suicide. The case manager immediately contacted Ms. L. and, after discussing the incident with her, determined she was not planning to commit suicide. The case manager developed a contract with Ms. L. who agreed that if she felt suicidal, she would contact the case manager immediately before she took any actions (Connecticut Community Care, Inc., 1991).

The ideal client caseload includes a mix of clients ranging from those requiring scheduled contacts to those requiring intensive case manager intervention. If all clients require intensive intervention, the case manager will have difficulty adequately managing the caseload, and may become vulnerable to burnout because of her inability to perform the case management role. In addition, these clients may have very high care costs because the case manager has not had time to deal with the problem before it became a crisis, or because she simply placed services rather than try to fully assess and resolve the problem.

One strategy used by case management organizations who care for very frail clients is to create interdisciplinary teams. The teams are composed of case managers with varying professional backgrounds, such as nursing, social work, gerontology, and counseling. These individuals contribute their unique discipline perspectives to problem resolution and to support of one another.

Documentation of Care Plan Changes

As noted in the previous chapter on Care Planning, documentation is an important aspect of the monitoring phase of case management. All contacts with the client, informed supporters, service providers, and others should be clearly documented in the client record. Documentation should include any care plan changes and the rationale for these changes.

Evaluation of the Care Plan

Client care plan evaluation involves measuring its effectiveness and progress toward meeting client care goals. Evaluation includes the following basic components:

- Are services being provided at the correct time in the prescribed amounts?
- Do provider reports document the client's status clearly?
- Are service providers billing for service accurately?

Other components of care plan evaluation include the impact of client outcomes and client satisfaction with services. The case manager should determine the impact of the care plan on client outcomes. The case manager evaluates the client in relation to client goals by obtaining feedback from the client, family, and service providers. For example, a client problem may be that she is unable to maintain desirable social contacts. The care plan goal is for the client to establish social contacts on a regular basis. Contacts could include telephone reassurance, a friendly visitor, or attendance at social gatherings. Care plan options could include friendly visitors, such as family, friends, neighbors, church members, volunteers, and companions; social gatherings, such as a family get-together, neighborhood activities, church activities, and adult day care program, a senior citizen group, and a support group; and, telephone reassurances by family, friends, neighbors, volunteer organization, church members, and formal provider agency service (Solan et al., 1986). The care plan is developed according to client choice and available resources. The case manager then can determine if the client has indeed established social contacts, and if the client is satisfied with the outcome.

The case manager evaluates whether the client's needs are being met, and if the client is satisfied with the services and care rendered. The case manager seeks feedback from the client, family, and service providers as indicated. If the client is not satisfied, the case manager should determine the reason for the client's dissatisfaction and take the indicated actions. Studies have shown that clients are generally reluctant to contact case managers and complain about services received. If the services are poor, the client will likely endure them silently for fear of losing the provider altogether (Solan et al., 1986). Compatibility between the service worker and the client can also be a key determinant in the client's satisfaction with provider services. Kane and Kane (1991) note that, "Clients would prefer adequate care from a worker they liked rather than excellent care from an unpleasant worker." In addition, the client's expectations may differ from what the worker can reasonably provide. It has been noted that elderly clients expect emotional support from their workers (Eustis & Fischer, 1991). The case manager can evaluate the information by visiting the client when the provider is also there and observing the provider's care firsthand. If the case manager has questions about the worker's care, the supervisor at the provider agency should be contacted and the worker's assigned tasks reviewed. If this review results in a change or clarification of the worker's tasks, the case manager should follow up with the client to make sure the changes have been implemented. The case manager should utilize client contacts to review her role in the client's care and make sure the client knows how to contact her and encourage her to call if there are any questions or problems.

The case manager evaluates whether the client's needs have changed, and if there are new problems that need attention. The ability of the informal caregivers to continue providing care should also be evaluated. The case manager again seeks feedback from the client, family, and service providers. Changes in a client's status rarely coincide with a scheduled monitoring contact or reassessment. The face-to-face reassessment visit provides an opportunity for an in-depth review and discussion of the client's status. For example, the case manager is dealing with a client experiencing confusion. The case management goal is to evaluate this problem. Evaluation options include medical and psychological evaluations. Subsequent service options to reduce or eliminate the confused state include follow up of medically ordered revision of prescribed medications or diet, mental health counseling, or family counseling. At the time of reassessment, the client was undergoing drug therapy and counseling to address the confusion. While the therapist noted improvement, both the client's supporters and case manager had had to deal with several incidents where the client's confusion left her in an unsafe situation. For instance, the client left her teapot on the stove and boiled it dry. At another time, the client left her apartment to refill her prescription, but after leaving forgot what her errand was and returned home without any medication. With these concerns in mind, the case manager talked with the client about temporarily altering her living arrangements until her confusion had lessened. The client's daughter visited daily, but was concerned about her mother's safety and was willing to have her mother move in with her until the situation improved. After much discussion, the client agreed to try this arrangement for a limited period.

Contract and Service Order Compliance

Provider contracts and service compliance can be both an administrative and a case manager responsibility. Administrative responsibility includes checking provider contracts against actual performance. Monitoring can be in the form of reviewing billings, staff training, provider reports, and other contractual obligations. Contract compliance is also verified through meetings with service providers. If the provider is having difficulty fulfilling contractual obligations, administrative staff will need to determine if the contract should be continued.

Developing Good Provider Relations

It is important to develop and maintain good provider relations. Several steps can be followed to foster positive provider relations. The case manager should clearly understand the provider's scope of practice and referral procedures, and whom she should contact for service questions.

Case management agencies and providers should encourage a joint participation in record audits, professional advisory committees, and educational programs. It is important for the case management staff to be viewed as competent and credible in their case management practice. Case managers also interact with physicians and should take the opportunity to discuss with them the role of case management in the care of their patients.

Furthermore, case management agency staff should be sensitive to the problems and difficulties faced by community service providers. Community service providers must cope with limited public funding. Service provider staff also face caseload pressures and may serve other, similar clients who do not have case managers. Thus, provider staff may find it difficult to accommodate case manager input on a client when in other situations they function independently. A provider may fail to report a problem or change in a client's situation, which can result in problems for the client and the case manager.

Community service providers may also not be accustomed to handling very difficult, long-term clients. Their typical client may receive services for a limited time period and must meet narrow eligibility definitions. The newer, less experienced staff may not be familiar with the subtle changes presented by a frail older person. The provider's assessment may be limited to a health focus, and they may not be as sensitive to the client's personality or family dynamics.

The politics of care also affect all community service providers, including case management agencies. Competition for scarce public and private funding may aggravate normally manageable "turf" issues between service providers and the case management agency. Cooperative relations among community service providers and the case management agency is always most advantageous to the client and strengthens the case for a community alternative to institutional care.

Other providers include individuals who are privately contracted by clients and families. Several studies have reported that clients frequently hire individuals to help them in specified areas before contacting a case management agency. In one study (Eustis & Fischer, 1991), nearly one-third of the clients had direct care workers not hired by the case management agency providing assistance. In the Channeling Demonstration (Carcagno et al., 1986), case managers found that, at initial assessment, 20% of the clients had already contracted privately with individuals to deliver certain services. According to these case managers, the private individuals proved to be valuable resources for care planning purposes as they were already familiar with the client's situation, were generally available for additional time, and could be trained for other tasks.

Quality Assurance

A basic expectation of service providers is that they deliver a quality service. The quality of services is compromised when the worker:

- is tardy or does not arrive to provide services at the client's home;
- fails to follow instructions or to complete assigned tasks;
- abuses the client; or,
- steals or damages the client's property. (Phillips, Applebaum, & Atchley, 1989)

If any of the above occur, the case management agency should determine: if this is reflective of the individual worker only or of the provider agency as a whole; if the staff are poorly trained or otherwise not qualified; if the provider agency is aware of the worker's actions; and, if the provider agency monitors its workers adequately.

The case management agency can review the provider's history of client complaints and the audited statements, and perform client/family satisfaction surveys.

It is important to note that the relationship formed between the client and the individual service provider is influenced by many factors. The worker may be privy to intimate details of the client's and family's situations. At times, it may be difficult to determine where the professional relationship ends and the personal one begins for both the client and the worker. While specific provider jobs are defined, such as homemaker service, workers often do extra tasks or stay at the client's home beyond the scheduled hours. As the lines between formal and informal blur, these workers perform additional services because they have developed personal, affective ties to the client (Eustis & Fischer, 1991). This type of relationship may cloud the client's objective assessment of the worker's service performance. The case manager must assist the client in the objective evaluation of the quality of the provided services. The case manager may list and define the tasks performed by the service provider. The case manager can make unscheduled home or site visits when the worker is there to personally observe the services provided. The client should be strongly encouraged to contact the case manager immediately if there is a problem with a service provider. The case manager should inform the client and family of the client's rights with regard to care.

The quality of long-term care services is a critical concern. Currently, there are no definitive national standards for provider services in home health care. A recent study, the Ohio Quality Assurance Demonstration project (Applebaum, Regan, & Woodruff, 1991), developed preliminary service guidelines. Quality assurance activities begin at the service delivery level and providers must take the primary responsibility for delivering quality care. Clients receiving long-term care services have unique, multiple needs and may interpret the quality of their care in different ways. If services are rigidly standardized, unique client needs may not be addressed and the quality of care may be undermined from the client's perspective. Another study, reported by the Hastings Center (Collopy et al., 1990), suggested that the imposition of rigid standards upon home care providers by regulatory agencies limited the professional discretion of agency workers. Flexibility is an important element in dealing with the complex and sometimes unpredictable challenges of the frail elderly. Excessively rigid standards may only hinder the client's helpers. However, it is also important to have relevant quality standards in order to protect clients from "dangerous care."

7 Case Management Settings and Practice Models, Staff Qualifications, and Supervisory Functions

Each case management organization defines its model of clinical practice in relation to its mission and vested authority. This definition should include specific practice guidelines and the boundaries of the case manager's authority. This chapter examines case management models, staff qualifications, and supervisory functions.

CASE MANAGEMENT SETTINGS

Case management is practiced across a variety of settings. These settings are discussed below.

Freestanding Agency

The freestanding agency model has an autonomous governing body. The service provided is case management only. The agency does not provide any other direct in-home or community services. Because of the relatively recent recognition of the unique practice of case management, this type of agency must be creative in maintaining and expanding its sources of funding. One of the strengths of this model is the objectivity of the care planning process, as the case manager has no financial interest in the arrangement of specific services.

Special Unit in a Direct Service Agency Model

In this model, the case management unit is located in an agency that also provides direct services such as family counseling, home health aide, or homemaker or information and referral services. This model benefits from its established reputation in the community. The challenge for this type of agency is to provide case management services that are perceived as objective yet are compatible with the agency's direct service functions.

Special Unit-Institution or Multi-Function Agency Model

This type of case management model may be located in multiple sites, such as hospitals, homes for the aged, or multipurpose senior centers. This model also benefits from the sponsoring institution's established reputation and experience. In this setting, it is important for the unit to retain a separate identity from other institutional services in order to be viewed as a component of rather than subordinate to the services offered in the larger institution.

Consortium Model

A consortium model refers to a variety of agencies working cooperatively under shared governance. The case management program functions to help clients receive assistance through the consortium service-provider network. This case management model is strengthened by a broad support network and by operational freedoms that may be greater than each individual cooperating agency. If the consortium is not fully supported, however, the case management unit can lose authority, and its autonomy may be diminished.

Insurance Case Management Model

The insurance case management model provides case management services to beneficiaries insured with the company. The case management function is usually of short duration and is related to an acute medical event.

CASE MANAGEMENT PRACTICE MODELS

Case management can vary from a simple information/referral model to a complex, long-term care model. In broad terms, three types of practice (Cline, 1990) can be delineated as shown below.

Medical Care Case Management

Associated with the hospital discharge planning process, medical-care case management practice refers to the coordination of home health services immediately following hospital discharge. Clients are followed on a short-term basis during the transition period from acute illness to stabilized home care services.

Catastrophic Care Case Management

Catastrophic-care case management practice models are usually associated with an insurance company. In order to control costs and make efficient use of health services, an attempt is made to identify the high cost users as early as possible.

The case manager provides short-term service for high cost clients such as burn victims, head trauma victims, and spinal cord injury victims. In these situations, case management services are usually terminated after a specified period of time.

Long-Term Care Case Management

The long-term care case management model serves individuals with acute or chronic illnesses and coordinates health, social, and community support services. In this practice model, the case manager is engaged in a long-term relationship with the client and works to create a care plan that is efficient and cost-effective. Clients served by that model may include older adults, AIDS victims, developmentally disabled individuals, children with congenital defects, and others with permanent impairments, such as traumatic brain injurys.

In all of these practice models, the case manager may have varying levels of control over purchased services. The case manager's authority may vary from only being able to recommend a plan of care to being able to authorize and pay for services. Control over service dollars may include monies from waivered Medicare or Medicaid programs, Older Americans Act funds, state appropriations, and private insurance benefits.

STAFF QUALIFICATIONS

Staff composition, qualifications, and numbers will vary depending on the organization's mission. The simple information/referral model will need fewer staff than the more expensive long-term care case management model. The remaining discussion will focus on the staffing needs for the long-term care case management model. The roles of the case manager, case manager assistant, supervisor, and support staff are explored.

Case Managers

Effective case managers must bc independent, self-motivated, and self-directed in their roles. They must be able to establish their own priorities and arrange their work schedules within organizational guidelines. The long-term care case management model is most likely to be serving frail elderly clients. Other case manager qualities are patience, acceptance, tolerance, respect, and nonjudgment. Case managers must be flexible in their attitudes and responsive to the older adult's wishes (Austin, 1983).

The National Council on Aging's Care Management Standards (NCOA, 1988) define the professional qualifications of the case manager as follows:

- Graduate of an accredited four year college or university with a degree in nursing, social service, gerontology, health, or other related area, with a minimum of two years of experience in a human service field; or,
- Graduate of a master's level professional program with a degree in social work or nursing, with one year of experience in a human service field.

Even with these professional credentials, the new case manager needs extensive orientation to prepare for the position. Unless the individual has had similar case management experience, no academic or other previous clinical experience can fully prepare the individual for the demands of the multiple tasks of case management. In addition to managing the comprehensive assessment, developing care plans, and arranging, coordinating, and monitoring services, there is the stress of dealing with a frail client population. At Connecticut Community Care, Inc., every case manager goes through six weeks of intensive orientation to every phase of the case management process before beginning full caseload responsibilities. It generally takes from six months to one year before a new case manager is effectively handling a full caseload.

The clinical practice of case management is professionally challenging and personally rewarding. The case manager with a high level of professional training is better prepared to view a client holistically and to skillfully assist the client through the fragmented health and community service systems. Through education in comprehensive assessment techniques, the case manager will be assisted in identifying the source of a client's problem and not just treating the symptoms. Finally, community care itself is a challenge, because it differs so radically from institutional care. Work is conducted outside of the protective auspices of an institutional setting. In addition to clinical skills, the case manager must develop expert knowledge about all available health and social services, and financial resources. The case manager must be committed to the client's right to self-determination. Because the client is in her home and not in an institution, she has the ultimate authority to decide and to control what services are to be provided in her home. Similarly, the case manager recognizes that she is an invited guest in the client's home. The case manager should be sensitive to the client's wishes about such issues as the scheduling of visits and to act with the client's informal supporters.

Organizations may employ either an individual or team approach to case management practice. In the former, one case manager has sole responsibility for clients, while in the latter two or more individuals, usually from different disciplines, work together. The advantages and disadvantages of both approaches are described below.

Individual Case Management Practice: The primary advantage to individual case management practice is that the client and her supporters have one contact for all of their concerns. The client and supporters develop and maintain a stable relationship with one case manager. This type of practice is best suited to a case management program with short-term, well-defined goals, where case managers do not become involved in complex client situations requiring significant amounts of their time. One of the major disadvantages of individual case management practice is that it can be professionally isolating. Case managers, if they are managing clients with complicated problems, may not have ready access to collaboration with their peers.

Team Case Management Practice: In the team approach to case management, a group of professionals representing different disciplines usually works together. Teams may be composed of nurses, social workers, physicians, psychologists, physical therapists, nutritionists, lawyers, conservators, and others. The usual team composition consists of social service personnel and nurses. One team member usually takes primary responsibility for the client's plan of care, and the others act as consultants and advisors to the primary case manager as needed. A major advantage of this type of practice is that the individual case manager accesses additional resources through the team interaction, and this allows the case manager to develop a broader perspective of the client's situation. Case managers can rely on team members in times of stress, minimizing possible burnout and improving morale. With team members available to substitute for one another in emergencies or when the primary case manager is ill, the client is assured of 24-hour coverage and a continuity of service by a person knowledgeable about her situation.

The Channeling Demonstration (Applebaum & Wilson, 1988), which targeted very frail older adults, reported several advantages to using the team approach in case management. Case managers who were not nurses reported the need for more information on medical procedures and on health conditions affecting clients. This knowledge helped improve communication with physicians, hospitals, and home health agency nurses. All staff requested additional information about cognitive impairments and mental disorders, and about how to work with clients with these problems.

Case Manager Assistant

The case manager assistant works with clients, families, service providers, and other internal agency staff to assist the case manager in the day-to-day management of the client caseload. Qualifications for the job may include having a high school diploma plus experience in the human service field. The case manager assistant performs many non-clinical tasks to support the case manager. Duties can include ordering nonmedical home care services, monitoring clients via telephone or home visit, assisting clients with entitlement applications, completing forms, and scheduling assessments, reassessments, and reviews. Some case manager assistants may be trained to handle prescreening and referral tasks. All case assistant duties are performed under the direction of a case manager.

Case Manager Supervisor

The case manager supervisor has been described as the essential provider of a supportive and consultative environment for the case managers (Applebaum and Wilson, 1988). The ideal supervisor possesses personal qualities similar to the case manager and acts as a teacher, clinical resource, and administrator. The National Council on Aging's Care Management Standards (NCOA, 1988) recommend:

- A minimum of a bachelor's degree in nursing, social services, gerontology, or other related field, as well as two years of relevant case manager experience; or, a master's level degreed professional with experience in gerontology or a related field, and two years of case management experience.
- Both professionals must have demonstrated an expert ability in the care manager role.

One of the supervisor's roles is to function as the voice for the case management staff with other administrative staff by expressing their concerns, problems, and needs. To be effective, the supervisor must respect the case managers under her direction and be empathetic to their needs.

The case manager supervisor's roles include assisting the case manager with clinical and stress management issues. As a teacher, the supervisor assists case managers in their ongoing growth and development. The supervisor provides advice on assessment, care planning, monitoring, and reassessment activities as needed. For instance, a supervisor might arrange for a joint assessment visit by a novice with an experienced case manager. The supervisor is aware of the history and problems of many of the clients served by the agency. Non-nurse case managers may be unfamiliar with geriatric health problems and need extra guidance from a nurse supervisor. A social worker supervisor is available to help case managers in negotiations with informal caregivers and formal service providers.

Also, case managers may experience job-related stress which usually occurs in two areas: clients service and time management. The case manager may be responsible for very frail, very dependent clients. These clients have significant service needs, demanding frequent monitoring, adjustment of care plans, and sometimes crisis intervention and management. Additionally, these clients experience high morbidity and high mortality rates. Informal caregivers may also be overburdened and have difficulties coping with the client situation. The case manager may need extra support in managing these daily stresses.

Time management issues may be another concern. Client caseloads may vary from 30 to 80 clients per case manager. In the Channeling Demonstration, case managers had client caseloads of 45 to 55 clients each, because of the clients' extremely frail natures. Twenty-two percent of the clients were unable to perform five Activities of Daily Living (ADLS), and most clients averaged two to three ADL deficiencies (Applebaum & Wilson, 1988). Juggling the demands of all of these clients could result in significant stress for the case managers.

The supervisor has several options in assisting case managers in job related stress. The supervisor may relieve the case manager of some client responsibilities and have her participate in such activities as attending professional educational conferences, special projects, or service training. These activities can provide the case manager with needed respite. If the case manager is particularly overburdened, the supervisor may arrange for temporary assistance. Inexperienced case managers often need assistance in learning how to manage their time. The supervisor may assist the new case manager by showing her how to develop a monthly planning calendar that includes scheduled assessments, reassessments, and monthly monitoring contacts. During a new case manager's orientation period, the supervisor should plan to schedule regular meetings, usually weekly, to review her activities and discuss any concerns. The supervisor is responsible for recognizing case managers who are experiencing work-related stress and assisting them in a stress management plan.

Each case manager has a specific need for supervisory assistance which is dependent on her professional background and previous experience. Supervisors are usually responsible for the clinical orientation of new case managers. In order to encourage creativity and problem-solving skills, the supervisor should avoid extensive directives to new case managers. The supervisor may encourage team building and support by meeting regularly with groups of case managers. In a case management team structure, the supervisor attends team meetings and provides guidance as indicated in resolving different client situations.

It is important to recognize that case managers require ongoing professional development. Case managers should participate in identifying their educational needs. The supervisor then may arrange an in-service program and should consider providing the active involvement of the most experienced case managers. Topics may be related clinical skills or community resources, providing extra stimulation for experienced case managers by allowing them to share their knowledge and enhance their public speaking skills.

Evaluation of case management practice is a critical component of the supervisor's role. The following areas of case management practice should be evaluated.

- ability of the case manager to explain case management and the agency's various programs to clients and caregivers
- accuracy in determining client eligibility for programs
- ability to educate and inform clients and families about choices and options for care
- effectiveness in interviewing skills in the assessment and reassessment process
- appropriateness of clinical skills in case management practice
- ability to develop appropriate care plans which include realistic client-centered goals, mobilization of the informal caregivers and formal providers, and creative use of resources
- ability to utilize all available reimbursement sources to fund client care plans
- documentation skills
- work behavior that includes understanding and support of agency policies, flexibility in accepting assignments, and effective use of interpersonal communication skills
- interest and involvement in their own professional development
- ability to develop goals for future practice

In summary, the supervisory role in a case management organization is a challenging one. The supervisor must be a teacher, a clinician, and an effective administrator.

Time and Caseload Management: The supervisor's administrative skills include caseload management. Supervisors play a key role in communicating agency policies and contractural responsibilities to the case management staff. The supervisor has significant responsibility in assuring that the case mangers are effectively meeting client needs and contractural responsibilities.

Crisis Management: Crisis management is an integral part of any organization's experience. Supervisors frequently represent the organization's administrative structure in the first response to client-related crisis. These crises may involve difficult ethical dilemmas, such as the client's right to self-determination versus safety concerns, conservatorship decisions, or institutionalization. These issues usually require extensive discussion with clients, all those involved with the client's care, the case manager, and agency administrative staff. The supervisor must facilitate resolution of these dilemmas, so that appropriate decisions are made. The supervisor often plays a key role in facilitating the resolution of these dilemmas. The supervisor acts as a role model for the new case manager who is making the transition from a traditional role to the case manager role. For instance, nursing staff who have provided direct client care may find it difficult to refer the client for ongoing nursing care. Social workers involved in ongoing client counseling must now refer the client to others for ongoing counseling.

Finally, the case management supervisor may be responsible for the overall management of program service funds. This activity may require allocation of resources to specific client caseloads and sometimes even to individual clients.

Administrative Support Services

Other administrative support services, such as support staff and the organization's management information system, also contribute to the effectiveness and efficiency of case management services.

Support staff: Depending upon the organizational structure, a case management agency may employ various levels of support staff. The following examples of support staff roles have carefully defined tasks that supplement case management services.

Intake specialist: The intake specialist accepts referrals for all programs offered by the agency. This individual provides callers with information about the case management program, screens for program eligibility, and refers people to other community resources when appropriate. This key staff position is often the first point of contact for the individual who is calling, and the intake specialist must have excellent communication skills.

Data entry operator: The data entry operator performs all duties related to data entry, such as input of information collected during initial client assessment and reassessment, of client service orders, of billing information, and of other pertinent data.

Medical transcriptionist: The medical transcriptionist is responsible for typing client records, including client history, modified physical examination, client profile, problem list, and progress notes. In addition, this individual types all client-related correspondence, and performs other assignments on request.

Team clerk: The team clerk maintains the client record systems by means such as updating the master list of clients, maintaining client clinical records, and assisting with preparing reports.

Per diem case manager: The agency may have the need for per diem case managers during summer vacations or times of high levels of new client admissions. The per diem case manager assists with regularly scheduled client follow-up activity. She should meet all applicable qualifications for a regular case manager and receive relevant orientation and supervision.

Management Information Systems

Effective management information systems generate information for use by both administrators and case managers.

The particular agency's needs will define the type of equipment and software necessary for the system. Administrative information needed includes agency financial reports, client statistical information, provider service costs, and case management service costs. Case manager time and activity reports assist supervisors in arranging client assignments. Case managers should receive feedback on relevant client information.

Administrators use the management information system to assist them in managing their business operation. Two key systems are the management system and the client system.

The management system includes the general ledger, the vendor system, and the employee payroll system. Case manager statistics, such as time spent with client- and non-client-related activity, is also an important component of this system.

Other relevant administrative reports may include monthly client census statistics, client assessment/reassessment data, claims data, and other program activities. The need for data integrity and client confidentiality is essential.

Supervisors and case managers also have data needs. The supervisor may use client data to help plan for staffing. For example, allocation of staff time may be enhanced by clients' reports of their places of residence. A report that documented waiting-list sizes for specific programs might indicate future staffing needs.

Data may assist case managers in their clinical role. For example, each case manager might have a report listing active clients with their telephone numbers. Such a report could provide an emergency list for use by all staff in case a client needed immediate assistance. Case manager efficiency is enhanced by reproduction of existing service orders. When services are adjusted, renewed, or terminated, these changes could be made without writing a new service order, saving the case manager valuable time and paperwork. Finally, reproduction of the most recent reassessment instrument allows the case manager to review the client's prior status during the course of the reassessment visit.

Learning packages could also be developed for case managers. For example, simulated client crises may help refine decision-making skills for experienced case managers, and simulated assessment visits may help new case managers develop their problem identification skills. Other training materials could include packages for documentation skills, negotiating and care planning techniques, contracting with clients and families to clarify care plan responsibilities, studying ethical issues related to long-term care, and conservatorship procedures.

In conclusion, the practice of quality case management in long-term care is complex. Case management, a recent practice model, is evolving. Lessons learned from these different practice models should contribute to the future refinement and understanding of the role and value of case management.

References

Applebaum, R., & Austin, C. (1990). *Long-term care case management: Design and evaluation.* New York: Springer Publishing Co.

Applebaum, R., Regan, S., & Woodruff, L. (1991). *Monitoring in-home supportive services: A report on Ohio's quality assurance demonstration.* Oxford, OH: Scripps Gerontology Center, Miami University.

Applebaum, R., & Wilson, N. (1988). Training needs for providing case management for the long-term care client: Lessons from the National Channeling Demonstration. *The Gerontologist, 28,* 172–176.

Austin, C.D. (Winter, 1983). Case management in long-term care: Options and opportunitis. *Health and Social Work, 8,* 16–30.

Barthel, D. W., & Mahoney, F. I. (1965). Functional evaluation: The Barthel Index. ARCH physicians medical rehabilitation, 1979. *Maryland State Medical Journal, 14,* 61–65.

Berk, M. L., & Bernstein, A. (1985). Use of home health services: Some findings from the national medical care expenditure survey. *Home Health Care Services Quarterly, 6(1)*, 13–23.

Berman, H. J. (1987). Adult children and their parents: Irredeemable obligation and irreplaceable loss. Bobrof, R. (Ed.). *Gerontological social work with families: A guide to practice issues and service delivery,* New York: The Haworth Press.

Brostoff, P. M. (1988). Ethical dilemmas facing private geriatric case managers. In Fisher, K., & Weisman, E. (Eds.). *Case manage-*

ment: Guiding patients through the health care maze: Perspectives, models, and practical considerations. Chicago, IL: Joint Commission on Accreditation of Health Care Organizations.

Bulcroft, K., Keilkopf, M. R., & Tripp, K. (1991). Elderly wards and their legal guardians: Analysis of county probate records in Ohio and Washington. *The Gerontologist, 31,* 156–164.

Cantor, M. (1991). Family and community: Changing roles in an aging society. *The Gerontologist, 31,* 337–346.

Capitman, J. A., Haskins, B., & Berstein, J. (1986). Case management approaches in coordinated community oriented long-term care demonstrations. *The Gerontologist, 26,* 398–404.

Carcagno, G. J., Applebaum, R., Christianson, J., Phillips, B., & Thornton, C. (1986). *The evaluation of the national long-term care demonstration: The planning and operational experience of the channeling projects.* Princeton, NJ: Mathematics Policy Research, Inc.

Carter, W. B., Bobbitt, R. A., Bergner, M., & Gilson, B. S. (1976). Validation of an interval scaling: The Sickness Impact Profile. *Health Services Research, 11,* 516–528.

Christianson, J. B., & Stephens, S .A. (1986). *Informal care to the impaired elderly: Report of the national long-term care channeling demonstration of informal caregivers,* Princeton, NJ, Mathematics Policy Research, Inc.

Clark, P. G. (1991). Ethical dimensions of quality of life in aging: Autonomy versus collectivism in the United States and Canada. *The Gerontologist, 31,* 631–639.

Cline, B. G. (1990). Case management: Organizational models and administrative methods. *Caring,* 9(7), 14–18.

Collopy, B., Dubler, N., & Zuckerman, C. (1990). The ethics of home care: Automony and accommodation. *The Hastings Center Report, 20,* 1–15.

Connecticut Community Care, Inc. (1985). [Client histories: Evelyn, Sophy.] Unpublished raw data.

Connecticut Community Care, Inc., (1991). [Case Management Institute.] Unpublished raw data.

Connecticut Community Care, Inc. (1991). [Client histories: Margaret, Alice, Sally, Mary, John, Ms. A., Dolly T., Ms. L., Jody.] Unpublished raw data.

Connecticut Community Care, Inc. (1991). *Reassessment instrument.* Bristol, CT.

Duke University Center for the Study of Aging and Human Development. (1978). *Methodology: Multidimensional functional assessment questionnaire.* (2nd ed.) Durham, NC: Author.

Estes, C. L. (1985). The United States: Long-term care and federal policy. *Home Health Care Services Quarterly, 6(4),* 315–328.

Eustis, N. N., & Fischer, L. R. (1991). Relationship between home care clients and their workers: Implications for quality of care. *The Gerontologist, 31,* 447–456.

Folstein, M. F., Folstein, S., & McHugh, P. R. (1975). Mini-mental state: A practical method for grading the cognitive state of patients for the clinician. *Journal of Psychiatric Research, 12,* 189–198.

Furniss, W. (1990). *Supervision of community-based case management.* Unpublished manuscript at Connecticut Community Care, Inc., Bristol, CT.

Gonyea, J. G. (1987). The family and dependency: Factors associated with institutional decision making. In Dobrof, R. (Ed.). *Gerontological social work with families: A guide to practice issues and service delivery* (pp. 61–73). New York, NY: The Haworth Press.

Greenberg, J., & Levitz, W. (1984). A basic strategy for financing long-term care. *Hospital Progress, 65(2),* 46–49, 72.

Grisham, M., White, M., & Miller, L. (1983). Case management as a problem-solving strategy. *Pride Institute Journal of Long-Term Home Health Care, 2(4),* 21–28.

Gurland, B., Kuriansky, J., Sharpe, L., Simon, R., Stiller, P., and Birkett, P. (1977). The comprehensive assessment and referral evaluation (CARE). Rationale, development and reliability: Part II.A factor analysis. *International Journal of Aging and Human Development, 8,* 9–42.

Hollman, F. (1989). United States population estimates by age, sex, race, and Hispanic origin: 1989. *Current Population Reports,* Series P-25, No. 1057, U.S. Department of Commerce, Bureau of the Census. Washington, DC: U.S. Government Printing Office.

Hughes, C. P, Berg, L., Danziger, Coben, L. A., & Martin, R. L. (1982). Clinical dementia rating scale. *British Journal of Psychiatry, 140,* 566–572.

Hutton, J. T., Dippel, R. L., Lowenson, R. D., Mortimer, J. A., & Christians, B. L. (1985). Predictors of nursing home placement of patients with Alzheimer's disease. *Texas Medicine, 81,* 41–43.

Issac, B., & Kennie, A. T. (1973). The set test as an aid to the detection of dementia in old people. *British Journal of Psychiatry, 132,* 467–470.

Jacobs J. W., Bernhard, M. R., Delgado, A, & Strain, J. J. (1977). Cognitive capacity screen: Screening for organic mental syndromes in the medically ill. *Annals of Internal Medicine, 86,* 40–46.

Kahn, R. L., & Goldfarb, A. I. (1960). Brief objective measures for determination of mental status in the aged (MSQ). *American Journal of Psychiatry, 117,* 326–328.

Kane, R. (1988). Case management: Ethical pitfalls on the road to high quality managed care. In Fisher, K., & Weisman, E. (Eds.). *Case management: Guiding patients throught the health care maze: Perspectives, models and practical considerations.* Chicago, IL: Joint Commission on Accreditation of Health Care Organizations.

Kane, R., & Kane, R. (1991, March). *Reassessing the state of geriatric assessment.* Paper presented at the American Society on Aging Meeting, New Orleans, LA.

Kapp, M. B. (1991). Health care decision making by the elderly: I get by with a little help from my family. *The Gerontologist, 3,* 619–623.

Katz, S., Ford, A. B., & Moskowitz, R. W., (1963). *Activities of daily living scale.*

Katz, S., Ford, A .B., Moskowitz, R. W., Jackson, B. A., & Jaffee, M. W. (1963). Studies of illness in the aged: The index of ADL. JAMA, *185,* 914–919.

Kemper, P., Applebaum, R., & Harrigan, M. (1987). *A systematic comparison of community care demonstratons.* Institute for Research on Poverty, Special Report Series: University of Wisconsin, Madison. Madison, WI: University of Wisconsin.

Kissick, W. (1970). Health policy directions for the 1970's. *New England Journal of Medicine, 282,* 1343–1354.

Kover, M. G. (1986). Expenditures for the medical care of elderly people living in the community in 1980. *The Millbank Quarterly, 64(1),* 100–132.

Lawlor, E. F. (1990). *The Public Policy and Aging Report.* Chicago, IL: Policy Research Association, Inc.

Lawton M. P., & Brody E. M. (1969). Assessment of older people: Self maintaining and instrumental activities of daily living. *The Gerontologist, 9,* 179–186.

Lieberman, M. A. & Kramer, J. H. (1991). Factors affecting decisions to institutionalize demented elderly. *The Gerontologist, 31*, 371–374.

Morris, J. N., Sherwood, S., & Mor, V. (1984). Hebrew rehabilitation center for the aged vulnerability index. An assessment tool for use in identifying functionally vulnerable persons in the community. *The Gerontologist, 24,* 373–379.

National Institute on Community-based, Long-term Care, affiliate to the National Council on the Aging, Inc. [NCOA]. (1988). *Care management standards: Guidelines for practice.* Washington, DC: Author.

Ostercamp, L. (1988). Family caregivers: America's primary long term care resource. *Aging, 358,* 2–5.

U. S. Department of Health, Education and Welfare [U.S. DHEW]. (1978). *PACE Assessment Instrument* (Working document on patient care management). Washington, DC: U.S. Government Printing Office.

Palley, A., & Oktay, J. S. (1989). Issues in setting the agenda for a long-term care policy for the frail elderly. *Home Health Care Services Quarterly, 10(3/4),* 15–43.

U.S. Department of Health and Human Services [U.S. DHHS]. (1987). *Personnel for health needs of the elderly through the year 2020.* (Report to Congress, September, 1987). Bethesda, MD: Author.

Pfeffer, R. I., Kurosaki, T. T., Harran, C. H., Chance, J. M., & Filos, S. (1982). Measurement of functional activities in older adults in the community. *Journal of Gerontology, 37(3),* 323–329.

Pfeiffer, E. (1975). A short portable mental status questionnaire for the assessment of organic brain deficit in elderly patients. *Journal of the American Geriatrics Society, 23,* 433–441.

Phillips, P. D., Applebaum, R., & Atchley, S. J. (1989). Assuring the quality of home delivered long-term care: The Ohio quality assurance project. *Home Health Care Services Quarterly, 10(3/4),* 45–65.

Population Reference Bureau, Inc. (1990). *America in the 21st century: Social and economic support systems.* Washington, D.C.: Author.

Quinn, J. L. (1986). Seeking quality alternatives in community-based programs. *Business and Health, 3(8),* 21–24.

Randall, D. A. (1989). Patient rights and provider accountability. *Pride Institute Journal of Long-Term Home Health Care, 8(2),* 4–10.

Reisberg, B., Ferris, S. H., Deleon, M. J. (1982). The global deterioration scale for assessment of primary degenerative dementia. *American Journal of Psychiatry, 139,* 1136–1139.

Reisberg, B., Ferris, S. H., & Franssen, E. (1985). An ordinal functional assessment tool for Alzheimer's type dementia, *Hospital Community Psychiatry, 36,* 593–595.

Rivlin, A., Weiner, J. M., Henley, R., & Spence, D. (1988). *Caring for the disabled elderly: Who Will Pay?.* Washington, DC: The Brookings Institution.

Robinson, B. C. (1983). Validation of a caregiver strain index. *Journal of Gerontology, 38,* 344–348.

Saluter, A. F. (1989). Marital status and living arrangements: March 1989. *Current Population Reports, Population Characteristics.* Series P-20, No. 445, U.S. Department of Commerce: Bureau of the Census.

Scharlach, A. E. (1988). *Survey of caregiving employees.* Los Angeles: TransAmerica Life Companies.

Selig, S., Tomlinson, T., & Hickey, T. (1991). Ethical dimensions of intergenerational reciprocity: Implications for practice. *The Gerontologist, 31,* 624–630.

Shapiro, E., & Tate, R. (1988). Who is really at risk of institutionalization? *The Gerontologist, 28,* 237–245.

Sharoff, B. (1983). TransAmerica community care organization: A broker model that worked. *Pride Institute Journal of Long-Term Home Health Care, 2(4),*

Shueman, S. A. (1988). A model of case management for mental health services. In Fisher, K. & Wessman, E. (Eds.). Case management: Guiding patients through the health care maze: Perspectives, models and practical considerations. Chicago, IL: Joint Commission on Accreditation of Health Care Organizations.

Solan, E., Granneman, M., Carter, E., Wells-Hunter, H., Decker, P., Bulvanski, S., Coleman, C., Kluxen, M., & Johnson, T. (1986). *National long-term channeling demonstration assessment and care planning for the frail elderly: A problem specific approach.* Philadelphia, PA: Temple University Institute on Aging.

Spitz, B., & Abramson, J. (1987). Competition, capitation and case management: Barriers to strategic reform. *The Millbank Quarterly, 65(3),* 348–370.

State of Connecticut (1987). *How will we pay?: Report of the gov-*

ernor's commission on private and public responsibillities for financing long-term care for the elderly. Hartford, CT: Author.

Sterthous, L. M. (1986). *Informal services and supports in the national long-term care channeling demonstration: A collection of practice oriented papers.* Philadelphia, PA: Temple University Institute on Aging.

Stevens, R., & Stevens, R. (1970). Medicaid: Anatomy of a dilemma. *Law and Contemporary Problems, 35,* 348–425.

Texas Technical University. (1985). *Functional rating scale for symptoms of dementia.*

Zung, W. W. K., (1965). A self-rating depression scale. *Archives of General Psychiatry, 12,* 63–70.

Index

Index